Picturing Health and Illness

Picturing Health and Illness
Images of Identity and Difference

Sander L. Gilman

The Johns Hopkins University Press
Baltimore and London

For Two Friends: Robert Michels and Roy Porter

Published in the United States of America by
The Johns Hopkins University Press
2715 North Charles Street
Baltimore, Maryland 21218–4319

Originally published in Great Britain by
Reaktion Books Ltd
as *Health and Illness: Images of Difference*

ISBN 0–8018–5197–1
LC 95–75700

A catalog record for this book is available from the British Library

Contents

Acknowledgements

I am grateful to Roy Porter for suggesting that this book be written. Versions of the chapters in it have been given as talks at Harvard, Cornell, the University of California at Davis, the Conference of the European Society for the History of Psychiatry and Psychoanalysis, and the Taniguchi Foundation Symposium on the History of Medicine. I wish to thank my editor at Reaktion, Michael R. Leaman, for his advice and help.

The sources for the images are to be found in the Photographic Acknowledgements. I am especially grateful to Lucy Keister and Jan Lazarus of the Historical Prints and Photographs collection of the National Library of Medicine in Bethesda, Maryland, for their help in this regard.

Alice was beginning to get very tired of sitting by her sister on the bank, and of having nothing to do: once or twice she had peeped into the book her sister was reading, but it had no pictures or conversations in it, 'and what is the use of a book', thought Alice, 'without pictures or conversations?'

Lewis Carroll, *Alice's Adventures in Wonderland*, 1865

1 How and Why do Historians of Medicine Use or Ignore Images in Writing their Histories?

The Typology of Illustrated Histories of Medicine

The question I want to address, at the beginning of this book on picturing illness and health, is why images, pictures, visual representations of all kinds have remained a stepchild in the writing of the history of medicine. In a real sense this book (and my own work) is an answer to this question, but the anxiety about the use of images needs explanation. Certainly there seem to be enough 'illustrated histories' of medicine to acknowledge the importance of images in the written history of medicine. And yet their function as part of the materials of medical history has always been peripheral at best. What can explain the anxiety of historians of medicine about the use of visual images?

Recently, the Oxford art historian Francis Haskell, following the lead of cultural and art historians as diverse as Michael Baxandall, Irving Lavin, Peter Paret, Theodore K. Rabb and Simon Schama, has again asked the important question of how and why cultural historians use visual images.[1] This questioning was in no small degree the result of the clear anxiety about the interpretability of such images in the work of an earlier generation of intellectual historians, who included, for example, Peter Gay.[2]

It is clear that chroniclers of cultural and social change have used images as material for their writing of history since the Renaissance. Drawing on the work of Arnaldo Momigliano, Haskell divides such writers into 'historians', whose work consisted and consists of spinning narratives, and 'antiquarians', whose work was collecting and cataloguing objects from the past, many of them images in one form or another.[3] In articulating the powerful need to reread these images from the standpoint of the narratives that are then spun about them, Haskell points out over and over again the danger of a misuse or suppression of images that would work against their correct meaning.

Embedded deeply in Haskell's sense of his own project as a historian, therefore, is the notion of the image that has a true as opposed to a false reading.[4] That, of course, compromises his analysis of the function to which historians have put the visual. In seeing each reading ('true' or 'false', 'right' or 'wrong') of an image as part of a chain of reading, in which each has an impact on and alters all subsequent readings, Haskell distorts the complex relationship between a sense of contemporary historical meaning projected into the past and the meaning attributed to visual representation in the past. This problem of the truth of visual sources haunts their use today. If read 'correctly' do they provide a window into the past or only the historian's projection of the visual culture of his own age into the reconstructed past?

Even after the work of Johan Huizinga, the figure who closes Haskell's study, using or not using or using visual sources 'incorrectly' remains a contentious undertaking. But this is to no little degree the result of a tautology of which Haskell is quite aware, for the visual arts in one form or another are part of the 'stuff' of cultural history. To ignore them or to 'misuse' them means to violate the presuppositions of writing 'cultural history' as a history of culture in the public sphere. This undertaking means that the visual is intrinsic to the definition of culture (either in its narrowest sense defined as 'high art' or in its broadest defined as 'human production').

The tautology that sees visual sources as a source to analyse visual culture has not generally been a stricture on the writing of the history of medicine. For the visual culture of medicine has not been seen as intrinsic to its 'stuff' either in its narrowest sense as the study of 'art/ artist and medicine' or in its broadest meaning incorporating all of 'the visual culture of medicine'. The visual arts have only a very ancillary relationship to the traditional definition of medical history as evolved at the turn of the century. Haskell himself ironically recapitulates this marginality in his introduction when he comments on the central problem of his book, his critique of 'some great historians for not having paid enough attention to the arts and . . . explicitly criticizing others for having done so in an unconvincing manner'. He observes: 'The historian of medicine is not expected to be able to cure a stomach ache: should the historian of a particular historical method be required to solve the problems raised by its use? . . . The aim of the chapters that follow is to explore how, when and why historians have tried to recapture the past, or at least a sense of the past, by adopting the infinitely seductive course of looking at the image the past has left of itself' (p. 9). Historians of medicine, according to Haskell's logic, are not physicians, but, according to his logic, they are also not cultural historians. It is precisely that historians of medicine *are* cultural historians and that the culture of medicine is as heavily involved with visual culture as any other aspect of modern cultural history that makes the anxiety about the use of the visual image in the history of medicine into a meaningful problem. Haskell's problem is the use and abuse of the visual image; it is also a problem for the medical historian.

Haskell's own study does not make overt reference to the visual culture of medicine. Yet he is concerned with the development of the relationship between appearance and character from the physiognomist Giovan Vincenzo Della Porta in the Renaissance through Johann Kaspar Lavater in the eighteenth century to the historian Jacob Burckhardt in the nineteenth century. The fact that Della Porta and Lavater rooted their theories in 'medical' models, models that defined somatic and psychological (or at least characterological) pathologies, which had their antecedents as far back as the semiotics of Hippocrates, is not evident in reading Haskell's discussion. And the reason for this is that the visual culture of medicine has been obscured by the very writing of medical history. When we turn to the history of medicine for our models of the use of visual materials, four overlapping typologies for images can be found, typologies that bridge the gap between Momigliano's 'historians' and 'antiquarians'.

In re-viewing the illustrated histories of medicine or those histories of medicine that use visual images, the four major roles of visual images for historians of medicine seem to divide nicely between the 'antiquarian' and the 'historical'. The 'antiquarians' use them as illustrations and as representations of facts about the real world, while the 'historians' use them as documents to show a self-contained visual language or iconography concerning health and illness that exist in specific traditions of visual representation and as objects to access cultural fantasies about health, disease and the body. All of these roles overlap in one way or another in their presuppositions concerning the use of visual images. This typology in the writing of the history of medicine is one that certainly is not unique to the use of images in the writing of general history. But following Haskell's argument, it is important to note that for most historians of medicine through the close of the twentieth century, visual images are an untouched source material. Unlike Haskell's cultural historians, who may know that this resource is present and choose not to employ it, medical historians tend to avoid visual sources even where they could play a straightforward and simple role in supporting their arguments. The typology of the use of the images, therefore, reflects the limitations rather than the breadth of the medical historians' use of visual sources in their writing the history of health and disease.

Throughout this book I shall be using the term 'illness' as an overarching category. I shall use it primarily to represent physical and mental states that are understood in Western culture as pathological and 'dangerous' because of their life-threatening, stability-threatening or chronic nature. 'Disease' is the social construct that always provides the frame for an understanding of 'illness'. Thus these two terms necessarily overlap, though they can and will be separated for heuristic reasons in our discussion. 'Disease' is thus never a mere label; it always relates to the social construction of 'illness'. What the cause of that 'illness' is remains unspecified. It may be somatic or psychosomatic or, as is usually the case, a complex mixture of physical and psychic causes and/or symptoms.

'Disease' is seen in most of the traditional illustrated histories of medicine through the use of images as 'mere illustration'. This is the most common use of images in writing the history of medicine. Who has not enjoyed opening up such 'coffee-table' books? These books, from the widely read illustrated medical history of Felix Marti-Ibañez, which first appeared as a series in *MD* magazine addressed to physicians, to the most recent, packaged illustrated story of modern medicine, seem to use images as pictorial fillers.[5] Marti-Ibañez saw his goal to 'bring beauty and romance to Medicine and to make medical practice the epic adventure it ought to be. To do this, I realized, it would be necessary to inspire the physician with the saga of the "great doctors", . . . to enable him to look on the world around him through the eyes of an artist and on the world of medicine through the eyes of a human being' (p. xi). For him, 'the illustrations in the narrative text itself are kinetic in character, portraying events and persons *in action* rather than inanimate objects, and showing monuments not as dead, dusty ruins but as a dynamic part of the physician's daily life in each country and period' (p. xiv). This claim for an active mimesis does not require close commentary: 'Through the magic of word and image, of old iconography and modern photography, of historically reconstructed scenes painted especially for this book by famed artists, is created the majestic cavalcade, across the multi-coloured landscape of the ages, of shamans, magi, philosophers, hakims, physickers, investigators, teachers and space physicians, who fought prejudice and ignorance, malice and adversity, to help ailing mankind' (p. xv). Marti-Ibañez's own work and use of illustrative materials was itself heavily indebted to the massive, three-volume illustrated French history of medicine edited by Maxime Laignel-Lavastine (1946), which reflected much the same epistemological construction.[6]

Later illustrated histories seemed to rely on this model as the authoritative means of using illustrations to show the progress from earlier medical practice. Indeed, Marti-Ibañez's work is cited in at least one later illustrated history of medicine as a prime example of the literary work of the author/physician, along with Oliver Wendell Holmes and William Carlos Williams.[7] The intent of such histories of medicine is clearly stated. 'This book', according to Hero van Urk, Professor of Surgery at Rotterdam, in the forward to Duin and Sutcliffe, 'gives the facts to those of us in medicine who are looking for historical perspective; but it also provides excellent entertainment for the general as well as for the medical reader'.[8] Some of these illustrated histories literally do away with historical commentary, relying on the exemplary quality of images (and texts) to carry their message. Carmichael and Ratzan compile extracts from the history of medicine and parallel them with images from the period.[9] Reaching from pharaonic Egypt to the late twentieth century, these texts move from the purely medical to the cultural and literary; the images themselves from the realm of medical illustration to high art. The intent is clearly stated: 'the collective evidence of image and text reassuringly testifies to the evolution of medicine from magic and myth to scientific thought' (p. 11). No analysis of the images is given in the text; the images stand on the page as visual evocations of a mood or context.

The images in these histories of medicine represent an unmediated window into the world of medicine that seems to enable the mass reading market to observe the physician at work across the centuries. A large number of such titles exist and they are clearly aimed at a mass reading (or, perhaps better, viewing) market.[10] In the history of psychiatry and psychology, the primary English-language illustrated history is that written by A. A. Roback and Thomas Kiernan in 1969.[11] This is also true of the illustrated histories of nursing.[12] All of these studies 'find' images and scatter them through their histories like antiquarians discovering the remnants of the past.

Such antiquarian use of images as windows into the world of medicine harks back to Victorian popular illustrated books on the freakish aspects of the world of illness that in turn continued the early modern broadside traditions showing medical anomalies such as joined twins or unusual tumours. (This tradition does not end with the death of Victoria. Art Newman's 1988 handbook of medical curiosa is an unselfconscious collection of freaks and oddities clearly in this vein.[13]) Like them, the frame for each image, the caption or the text commenting on the image, seems only to replicate in words the content of the image used. The implication in all these images is a distance between the observed and the observer (whether physician or patient or potential patient). This distance may be articulated in terms of 'progress' from a primitive past or 'difference' from a pathology or physical anomaly. All of this is captured in the captions to the images. Indeed, the importance of the caption as a source of commentary is mentioned in at least one of these histories.[14] The illusion is of an unbroken gaze into the past that defines the positive or protected status of the observer. But it remains the unusual and the different that are still captured in these illustrated histories and their images. No better evocation of this can be found than Jim Harter's handbook of '4800 copyright-free engravings', all taken from nineteenth-century medical sources. Here page upon page of images intended for further reproduction represent the antiquarian image of medicine. Its intent is to 'recreate the world of medicine as it was in the past – by exploring in great detail all of the major areas of medicine and also a number of peripherally related subjects . . . [It is] an ultimate visual reference source for doctors, nurses, medical and anatomy students, people in the many health related fields, artists, designers, historians, lovers of Victoriana, and any one else having an interest in this fascinating area of human endeavor'. The end result is a visual handbook without any commentary whatsoever, a peep-show to be used to document the 'bizarre and pathological'.[15] And that is understood as being different in quality from the nature of the observer.

The twentieth-century continuation of this illustrative tradition has a clear ideological basis. By presenting an 'unmediated' (that is, uninterpreted) representation of health and illness, the quaint practices of the past are 'seen' by the reader cheek and jowl with portraits of the 'Great Men', the medical innovators of the past. In all of these heroic histories, a sense of the progress of medicine can be had by looking at the pictures. We, the lay viewers, can understand 'how far we have come' by our own observation of these illustrations. In the case of views of contemporary medicine, such as the thematic picture story by Smolan that surveys the state of present medical practice, the underlying assumption is of a high level of contemporary medical competency as opposed to the unviewed but clearly less than adequate practices of a fantasy 'yesterday'. Illustrations without overt analysis provide the intrinsic ability for viewers to measure the realities of medical change for themselves, or so it seems. The use of images of health and illness are tied to an ever-improving reality of medical care of the patient in this model.

Even such a naïve use of pictures of all types as illustrations is highly manipulative. It is clear that the selection or editing of the material to 'tell a story' means that the frame is a procrustean bed into which the image is fitted. What is often unstated is the overt closure implicit in the use of such images. The assumption is that the narrative is complete rather than partial (as all narratives must be) and that the images provide 'representative' or 'unmediated' access to the material world of the narrative. Such picture histories, however, employ an epistemology that assumes a relationship between the image and some reality external to the historian and the reader.

Such an uncommented 'window' into the past is linked closely to the epistemological basis for the second use of images in writing the history of medicine. This is the flipside of the work of Harter. Mechanical reproduction is vital here. The user of the image as illustration has no compunction about using any type of image to illustrate the progress of medicine, from the votive figures of Greek temples to the drawings of Andy Warhol. Thus in Helmut Vogt's history of the relationship between physician and patient (1984), which uses visual sources from the fifteenth to the twentieth century, the photograph is conscientiously avoided.[16] His intent is to record the antiquarian images and the attitudes documented in modern cartoons and caricatures. In contemporary 'historical' usage, older forms of mechanical reproduction, such as the engraving or the lithograph with their 'evident' aestheticization for the late twentieth-century observer, must give way to the photograph, a 'real' window into the realities of the past. As Joel-Peter Witkin writes in the introduction to a selection of historical medical photographs:

The work of painters and sculptors, regardless of content, must finally be presented as works of the imagination. It is only in our epoch that we possess the permanent mirror of memory we call photography, the most truthful representation of reality ever known. . . . The camera has given us the means of seeing ourselves in others, ourselves harmed, unloved, deformed, even dead. These images are triumphant contributions in the evolution of the quest for our highest attainment, to unselfishly help and heal one another, to eradicate all disease, both social and pathological.[17]

Once a naïve, mid-nineteenth-century positivistic genre expectation of the photograph as a mimetic reproduction of reality is introduced, there is a heightened sense that such images have a true 'proof' value, that is, they show you the way things really were.[18] Here, it is not that the image is an index to a present reality but rather that it permits the reader/viewer to open a window onto a past reality.

One answer to this view is that the image functions as a representation of power in the real world, such as explored in the work of Fox and Lawrence (1988) on British and American medical photographs.[19] They dismiss the earlier view that 'photographs, unlike hand-made pictures, invariably froze and copied an instant of reality', and understand that the photograph 'made it easier and cheaper to record and duplicate the sort of images which for centuries artists had made by hand' (p. 7). For Fox and Lawrence, the photograph comes to be the expression of contemporary aesthetic conventions. They stress the mimetic relationship of these conventions to the social and economic role played by the photograph in nineteenth- and twentieth-century cultural life. The photograph does not display life as it was, but rather the usually invisible lines of social power in the world of medicine. While they stress that photographs are not a 'privileged source' for the documentation of details (such as 'dress or artefacts'), they tend to see it as a privileged source for the social self-representation of medicine. While aware that the photograph does continue the traditions of other visual representations, they treat the photograph as attaining a higher degree of mimesis because of the qualities ascribed to it in the general visual culture.

As in the illustrated history, the image and the reality are one. But in the illustrated history, the illustrations echo the argument of the text; here the image is used as evidence for the historian's argument. In such images, the historian says to the reader/viewer: You can see the truth of my statement for yourself, as you too have this objective window into history as it really was. Let us however, the historian continues, be aware that these are images and that they also have a history. Such theories of the medical image enter into the very use of images in medical textbooks, especially those in psychiatry that have a strong historical component. Here the images claim to be a window on reality, even when they represent internal psychic states such as depression.[20] The captions to these photographs all serve as frames to draw the reader's attention to the meaning of the photograph, a meaning that may not be apparent on first viewing. These images are now not 'merely' illustrations of a lost world, but part of the claim for the truth of the historian's reconstruction of the world as it really was. This medical antiquarianism echoes the antiquarian's claim that the visual object is an unproblematic fragment of past reality.

The 'historians' of medicine use images in a more self-aware manner. Thus the third model for the use of images in the writing of the history of health and disease stresses the artistic medium itself and the internal iconographic tradition of the work of art. It is not the truth of the external world of medical practice and social reality that is evoked in this model, but rather the rules of artistic representation. Such studies are often not clearly labelled as histories of representations, and indeed seem to evoke a history of medical practice. Yet when they are examined they tend to be internal histories of medical representations. How well or poorly such images reveal the actual practices or beliefs of medicine is not an issue in these studies. Rather, it is the means by which the image is constructed – its internal vocabulary – that are central. Thus the short overview by Thornton and Reeves stresses the 'history of the development of medical book illustration [that] has been governed by the materials and techniques available'.[21] As in the work of Robert Herrlinger on the history of medical illustration, this emphasized the autonomous artistic vocabulary of the medical image.[22] An analogous view is to be found in the standard French study of the topic.[23] Medical iconography has been seen as separate from yet related to the general iconography of Western representational art following the guidelines laid down in the mid-nineteenth century by Ludwig Choulant's history of anatomical illustration and its relationship to high art.[24] The problem arises again when the contemporary medical historian wishes to turn to contemporary, non-representational art for images of internal, subjective states. Such studies of 'medicine and art' rarely extend beyond the bounds of the mimetic representations of illness and healing, no matter even if the cultures studied include non-Western visual traditions.[25] Francis Haskell shows how even semi-representational art can and has been used as a source for cultural historians. But such a reliance on representational art (i.e., art that provides a recognizable visual analogy to experiences in the world) in medical history makes such a movement difficult.

The study of the representation of medical subjects and especially psychiatric ones in 'high' art is closely related to this approach to the iconography of medicine. Most often such studies examine medically significant themes in high art as a means of examining the specific iconography of that topic. Rarely is there any concern about whether what is being presented is 'progressive' medicine or even 'real' medical practice, though this is often assumed. What is of importance is the language of the image. Here, the reality is that of the tradition of representation. The captions often are used to point to specific references or provide links among images.[26] Less frequently, the claim for a limited tradition of autonomous medical iconography is examined as separate from the greater art-historical one.[27] Specific studies of the relationship of given artists to specific themes in medicine also stress only the iconographic tradition.[28]

Similar to such historical studies from the world of high art are the histories of popular, medical caricature.[29] Here, it is medicine's representation in other contexts, such as politics, that is of interest. No claims are made about the truthfulness of the image as a window into the world of medicine. What is stressed here is the use of medical imagery as

the internal vocabulary of the images. Rather, the genre expectations of the work of art (for example, the link between caricature and visual irony) and the visual devices (such as exaggeration) that are its particular means of expression are central to such studies.

The fourth way of employing visual materials in the writing of the history of medicine is to make the image itself the subject of the analysis of cultural fantasies of health, disease, and the body. Here the image serves as a mirror of the self as formed by the fantasies of any given culture about illness and health, concepts themselves that are structured by notions of what the self is. Only recently have the best social historians of medicine, such as Charles Rosenberg, come to understand the theatrical function of illness as both an actor and the frame of the action.[30] In my own studies of the visual representation of both the mentally and somatically ill, I demonstrated the close relationship between representations of illness and cultural fantasies about illness.[31] This in no way undermined the reality of illness, including mental illness, but rather stressed the function that such a vocabulary of images has. One could access the world not of reality but of fantasy through the examination of representations of difference. These were 'real' cultural fantasies that could and did affect not only those who generated these images to represent and thus control the world, but also those who served as the objects of representation. The patient and the physician were both part of this system of cultural fantasy. Indeed, one could speak of a closed system of representation that shaped and was shaped by the needs of all of the social roles defined by the doctor–patient dyad. Work in this vein has been carried out on psychiatric images by Georges Didi-Huberman (1982) and Elaine Showalter (1985), and on somatic topics by Michael Fried (1987), Ludmilla Jordanova (1989) and Barbara Stafford (1992).[32] Recently Kathy Newman has applied these structures to a brilliant examination of images of wounded American Civil War soldiers and evolved a complex reading of the construction of the material body in pain.[33] In all cases it is the unseen component of the cultural fantasy that is made visible in these images through the work of the historian. We as readers are not shown the reality of daily life through images, but rather subjective and intersubjective realities.

One further category that is closely related to the image as representation of the fantasies of illness is the concern of historians with the tradition of visual creations made by the mentally ill. Following the work of Hans Prinzhorn (1886–1933) in the 1920s, studies of the art of the mentally ill provided images of the painters as well as their works of art. The captions related these images to an internal reality of mental illness made visible through the artistic process. Here the distinction between representational versus non-representational images in the history of psychiatry becomes unimportant. For such works always stress the universal, unconscious processes behind the overt images. One could therefore explicate non-representational images as a measure of internal states, and those images that evoked specific themes through some type of overt representation.[34] Individual studies of mentally ill artists tended to replicate such models of analysis.[35]

Recent work on the history of the art of the mentally ill has tended to move to a cultural contextualization of these images, and stress the ideological context of the collection and analysis of such works of art within the world of medicine.[36] In these historical studies, the reality to be captured was the cultural context of the nineteenth- and early twentieth-century fascination with the artistic production of the mentally ill. As in the study of medical themes in high and popular art, the analysis of the history of the art of the mentally ill stressed thematic as well as formal questions: What are the topics addressed in the art of the mentally ill? What are the means by which these topics are represented? These questions are identical to those raised by psychiatrists such as Prinzhorn, but their answers are sought in historical rather than psychological contexts. These studies also address the fascination of the pathological 'quality' ascribed to these works in warranting their collection and analysis. In studies of the history of the interest in the art of the mentally ill, the 'pathological' comes to be understood as a purely constructed category. These works thus position themselves against the presuppositions of earlier works on the subject. The overarching claim of such histories of the study of art of the mentally ill is that there are no specific internal realities to be examined, only the external world internalized and represented in this art. Again and again these studies of 'outsider' art relate this tradition to the visual vocabularies of high art.[37] Only very rarely has there been an attempt to provide a serious discussion of the art of the mentally ill with both internal (psychological) as well as external (historical) categories of analysis.[38] These questions and their attendant images are rarely included in even the most extensive histories of medicine.[39]

Each of these approaches to the use of images in the history of medicine needs specific types of images. And indeed, each reading can be quite correct in its specific tradition. What has heretofore been avoided is the idea of multiple, simultaneous meanings, the very ambiguity that is inherent to visual images, no matter what their venue. What has been lacking is a comprehensive sense of the function that images can have in the contemporary study of the history of health and illness as it is practiced today. Rarely does the historian of psychiatry turn to the wide spectrum of images and draw from their totality. What untold tales could these images spin if they were understood as connecting all of the models above – from the naïve attraction that picture books have for the reader, to the notion that the image can give us access to realities and fantasies of worlds past and present, to the view that works of art have rules by which they represent the world and that it is important to know what those rules are and how they function.

The multiple typology of the use of images to date raises three interlocking problems: Why the initial anxiety about images in the writing of the history of medicine, especially, psychiatry? What is the power of such images, especially images associated with madness, and why does Western culture have the need to create categories that control them? How do such images capture the historical fantasies about mental illness, even while serving as veridical sources for 'facts' about the treatment or status of the mentally ill and functioning within specific representational traditions?

The History of the Illustrated History of Medicine

To understand the development of the multiple and contradictory uses of images of health and illness in histories of medicine, one must return to the meaning of the visual image during the late nineteenth century. Two academic disciplines, the medical speciality of psychiatry and the academic speciality of the history of medicine, were created within two decades of one another. It is precisely in the period following Jakob Burckhardt's cultural history, according to Francis Haskell, that the visual became accepted material for the academic historian.[40] It is immediately evident that the new field of psychiatry needed to create a visual epistemology for itself parallel to that existing for the other medical sciences in the age of microscopy, bacteriology and radiology – all new sciences dominated by the visual image. See it and it is real.[41] Nineteenth-century academic psychiatry could and did call on an older tradition of physiognomically representing the mentally ill. These traditions also appear within the works of nineteenth-century academic cultural historians, such as Hippolyte Taine, as an appropriation of visual sources to gauge the character of the shapers of history.[42]

Moreover, the first practitioners of the new speciality of psychiatry in France were also the first popular historians of psychiatry. They needed to create a genealogy for their new science that was rooted in the status of the visual image as a delineator of 'real' scientific medicine as well as in the practice of cultural history in their day. Without a doubt the most important figure in this tradition was Jean-Martin Charcot (1825–93), the first Professor of Mental Diseases at the University of Paris (1872, Member of the Academy of Medicine and Professor of Pathological Anatomy; 1882, first chair-holder as Professor for Mental Illnesses), for whom the visual image had a special and important function.[43] But what is even more important is the link of the epistemology of the new 'science' of psychiatry in Paris to the popular history of mental illness. Proof was to be found of the visual categories and nosologies employed by late nineteenth-century psychiatry in visual analogies sought in the high arts. These 'historical' sources were captured and used through the new scientific means of reproducing images, photography and, later, film.[44]

In Charcot's conception, the realism of such images transcended the crudity of the spoken word. In a letter to Sigmund Freud of 23 November 1891 concerning the transcription of his own famed Tuesday lectures Charcot commented that 'the stenographer is not a photographer'.[45] It is the photographer who can best capture the 'reality' of mental illness; and if not the photographer, then at least the trained physician/artist. The combination of a notion of the positivism of 'science' with the prestige of the scientific practitioner gave these images their status as evidence. The means of reproduction is therefore as important as the iconography used in these images to provide a readable text for the trained interpreter. Having subconsciously established patterns of description rooted in classic iconographies of insanity, it was relatively easy to find these patterns replicated within the visual record of Western civilization. This became true even to the degree that the patients of such physicians learned an adequate visual vocabulary so as to reproduce the visual traditions from which the description of their illnesses stemmed.

The audience for Charcot's monographs, and for those of his major collaborator, Paul Richer (1849–1933), on the visual tradition of mental illness was not merely 'professional'.[46] Like the audience of his Tuesday lectures, the audience for his books was the educated middle class of Paris. Indeed, the professional audience for psychiatric literature was in the process of being created during the late nineteenth century. These books were aimed as much at the educated lay audience as at a professional medical/historical one. Such books provided a higher status for the new profession, as they placed it in a long history, and they showed the lay audience that the technical knowledge the new profession had to have to 'look at' and 'diagnose' various forms of mental illness were refinements of the high culture that defined the intellectual at the turn of the century.

The sort of image that Charcot and Richer use in their histories of mental illness and difference reflect the adaptation of a particular tradition of using images. It was in no way subtle. Part of it was accomplished by 'outlining'. Charcot provided skeletal outlines of works of art (of the sort that Freud enjoyed producing himself, as in his study of Michelangelo's Moses of 1914), which stressed precisely the attributes that Charcot wanted the reader to 'see'. This tradition harks back to the first French illustrated atlases of mental illness, such as that compiled by J.E.D. Esquirol at the beginning of the nineteenth century. With such outlines, historical images supposedly representing psychopathological states were made visually identical to images of contemporary patients representing the same type of actions and thus identical conditions. Thus in terms of their 'proof value' all these images were identical, and they also stood in a history of the gradual professionalization of the role of the psychiatrist after the French Revolution. Likewise, Paul Richer incorporated similar images in his own work.[47] These were presented as analogous to the visual tradition in art in other historical sources that also used such images as 'proof'. The German response to such a use of the image in writing a presentative history of psychiatry with its teleological goals being the truths of the new (in the late nineteenth century) French psychiatry can be judged in Freud's own response to this technique. Freud's training with Charcot was a training in seeing the patient and the signs and symptoms the patient exhibited as the key to diagnosis.[48] One can argue that Freud's intellectual as well as analytic development in the 1890s was a movement away from the 'meaning' of visual signs (a skill he ascribes to Charcot in his obituary of 1893) to verbal signs, from the crudity of seeing to the subtlety of hearing.[49] Freud's rejection of the visual, one might add, precipitated a general negative response within avant-garde psychiatry to the meaning of the visual as 'scientific evidence'.[50]

Charcot therefore established a set of explicit assumptions about images in the writing of the history of illness (illus. 1). For Charcot all illness – mental and physical – had a somatic dimension. Just as pathology in the body could be measured by physical signs, so too were psychopathological changes to be seen in or on the body. The link between the historical and contemporary image showed the reality of the unchangeable visual patterns of mental disorders over time. Ancient images of smallpox paralleled contemporary images; ancient images of hysteria must then parallel contemporary images. For Charcot, older images from high and popular art had validity as proof if their visual structures could be echoed in modern, high-tech media

2° Un tableau plus important encore sur le même sujet, au musée de Vienne;

3° L'esquisse pour le tableau précédent, au même musée;

4° Une gravure de Marinus, reproduisant avec quelques légères modifications le tableau de Vienne;

5° Une étude pour la tête de la *Possédée* du tableau de Vienne;

6° Un dessin dans les collections du Louvre ayant trait au même sujet;

7° Une gravure d'après un tableau inconnu représentant *saint François de Paul montant au ciel*, et dans lequel se trouvent au premier plan un homme et une femme possédés.

Il a fallu toute l'intuition du génie, jointe à une rare acuité d'observation, pour saisir et fixer avec tant d'effet et de sûreté les traits fondamentaux d'un tableau si changeant et si complexe. La figure de la possession créée par le pinceau de Rubens est un véritable type. Elle est en même temps une image si fidèle de la nature, que sous tous ses aspects elle demeure vraie, et que, aujourd'hui, à plus de deux siècles de distance, nous y surprenons les signes indéniables d'une affection nerveuse alors méconnue.

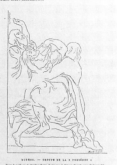

SAINTE CLAIRE DÉLIVRE UNE DAME DE PISE
D'après Adam Van Noort (XVI° siècle).

RUBENS. — GROUPE DE LA « POSSÉDÉE »
Dans le tableau de l'église Saint-Ambroise, à Gènes, d'après une photographie.

Nous n'aurons pas de peine à démontrer par l'étude de ces différentes œuvres, au point de vue qui nous retient, comme Rubens sut voir la nature et avec quel respect il sut la copier. Aucun maître n'a été plus injustement discuté sur sa conception du dessin.

Tel de ces possédés offre des caractères si vrais et si saisissants, que nous ne saurions rencontrer ou imaginer une représentation plus parfaite des crises que nous avons longuement décrites dans les ouvrages récents, et dont nos malades de la Salpêtrière nous offrent journellement des exemples typiques.

Nous allons passer en revue les différentes œuvres du maître anversois qui confirment nos remarques techniques en même temps que notre admiration.

Tableau de l'église Saint-Ambroise, à Gènes. — Les deux tableaux sur le même sujet de la guérison miraculeuse de la possession, celui de Gènes et celui de Vienne, auraient été exécutés la même année (1620), à quelques mois d'intervalle. Nous trouvons dans un travail de M. Paul Mantz sur Rubens quelques détails fort intéressants sur les circonstances de leur exécution.

CHARCOT ET RICHER. — Les démoniaques dans l'art.

1 'Historical' outlined illustrations (after Adam van Noort and Rubens) of hysteria, from Jean-Martin Charcot and Paul Richer, *Les démoniaques dans l'art* (Paris, 1887).

such as photography. From the invention of perspective to the development of the photograph, the innovations of Western art and science made the representation closer to the real world. And it is these images that can now be used as proof within the new science of psychiatry. For Charcot these images provided validity for his own means of diagnosing mental illness. And it was this validity that underwrote his claims for a new medical science – psychiatry – rooted in observable, experimental data and based in France. For it was not only as science, but French science, the science of Louis Pasteur and Claude Bernard, that Charcot had to justify his new speciality.

The close association between Charcot's theory of mental illness and his epistemological reliance on the process of visualization was part of the reason for the decline in the use of the image in medical historiography. With Charcot's unexpected death in 1893, his theories and methods underwent a sudden and rapid decline. Indeed the collected works of Charcot, begun as a monument to his memory, were quickly abandoned, and his method, particularly his reliance on visualization, became discredited in Paris, except among his personal disciples. It was they alone who continued the various projects of Charcot, projects that no longer played a substantial role in French or

European psychiatry. This rejection was to no little degree the result of the perceived superficiality of Charcot's somatic approach to mental illness, but it was also keyed to his mode of presenting visual evidence.

The response to the use of images in the German tradition in which the history of medicine as a discipline was founded was very different. Karl Friedrich Jakob Sudhoff (1853–1938) was the first Professor of the History of Medicine at Leipzig (1905) and *de facto* the creator of the modern academic discipline of the History of Medicine in Germany.[51] Trained as a physician, Sudhoff also studied history: in 1878 he was an assistant at the Charité under Rudolf Virchow while at the same time studying history with August Hirsch at the University of Berlin. In 1898, only five years after Charcot's death, he persuaded the German Association of Natural Scientists to add a section on the history of medicine and the natural sciences to their annual meeting. This movement eventually led to the professionalization of the discipline and the creation of the first chair in the history of medicine in Germany, which Sudhoff then held.

In Sudhoff's professionalization of the history of medicine, he used illustrated materials as the basis for his own idiosyncratic work in the history of syphilis, reproducing images of great interest and complexity. His images were often incidental illustrations from broadsides on the history of syphilis or the history of anatomy.[52] Certainly there was no attempt to write a history of either syphilis or the body based on the sixteenth-century visual sources that Sudhoff reproduced. Yet Sudhoff was sufficiently sophisticated about the history of media to believe strongly that all images (except for photographs) 'bring a subjective quality to the material examined or offered as proof, the appraisal of which in addition possesses a subjective evaluation in spite of the greatest accuracy and exactitude'.[53] This subjectivity is missing in the photograph, a medium he designates as a 'self-triggering photochemical process'. Thus the proof of the progress of medicine can lie in the development from earlier means of imagining the body, as in his work on the history of anatomical illustration, to the world of the photograph and the x-ray.[54] 'Subjective' images could, however, form the stuff of 'objective' history.

Sudhoff employed a version of the Rankean model of history – attempting to document the 'way it really was' in the Renaissance, but also drawing from the Renaissance meanings for his own time. The Renaissance and the Baroque, for German historians of the late nineteenth and early twentieth centuries, from Jacob Burckhardt to Walter Benjamin, were the self-constructed periods best able to support such a treatment. They were seen as distanced enough from the national cultures of the late nineteenth and early twentieth centuries to provide distinct categories separate from contemporary concerns and yet, like the nineteenth century, understood themselves as ages of secularization and science. For the struggle of 'theology' and 'science' is a central trope in the history of medicine in the late nineteenth century. It is of little surprise that Sudhoff's cultural hero, the figure to whom he devoted most of his scholarly work and energy, was Paracelsus.

Sudhoff's intention was to use the historical moment as a means of elucidating the present and prognosticating the future. In this he broke with the older view of the history of medicine advocated, for example, by Theodor Puschmann in 1889.[55] Puschmann had given a three-fold rationale for the writing of the history of medicine: to add to general education (*Bildung*), to establish professional knowledge, and to aid in the ethical education of the physician. In his inaugural lecture on Puschmann, held on 4 February 1906 in Leipzig, Sudhoff advocated that the historian of medicine should stop getting mired in multitudes of facts; rather, the historian should selfconsciously select those facts from the past that are important for the present.[56] Such a process of selection demanded an overview of the entirety of a field, but it was vital to interpret materials as well as present them. Thus Paracelsus, whose work came to be the centrepiece of Sudhoff's academic activities, becomes not only a figure from the past but a symbol of the ideal physician of the nineteenth century, struggling against a repressive conservative medical tradition. But the only one who can make the leap from fact to interpretation is the trained historian, not the physician. It is the new professional historian who provides meaning for facts and draws them into the present.

Yet the German historiographical tradition avoided the illustrated historical text. This set the writing of 'serious' history apart from anthropology, which in the late nineteenth century relied heavily on illustrated volumes. Serious, 'scientific' histories of medicine could reproduce illustrations but they could not acknowledge them as 'proofs' for any arguments. This practice continued in the work of historians of medicine like Sudhoff's student Henry Sigerist (1891–1957), who, like his teacher, was quite aware of the relationship between the history of art and the history of medicine, but never employed it in his own writing.[57] Only texts from the past could serve as proof. In Germany, 'serious' histories of medicine, such as that of Ernst Schwalbe, used in the teaching of the history of medicine to medical students, avoided illustrations of all types.[58]

Indeed, it was only in 1921 that Sudhoff and Theodor Meyer-

bekämpfung einen gewaltigen Ausschlag nach vorwärts aufwies. Bei der Pest des JUSTINIAN im 6. Jahrhundert, die die greulichsten Verheerungen machte, schweigt die ärztliche Literatur, und von Abwehrmaßregeln der Behörden ist keine Rede. Bei der Epidemie des schwarzen Todes werden schon zu Anfang vielfach scharfe Absperrungsmaßnahmen ergriffen, die sogar Teilerfolge brachten, und sofort setzt eine große Literatur in allen Ländern Europas ein. Mehrere hundert Pesttraktate sind allein in den letzten anderthalb Jahrhunderten des Mittelalters zu verzeichnen. Ja, in wenigen Jahrzehnten entwickelte sich in Italien und Südfrankreich ein Abwehrsystem mit

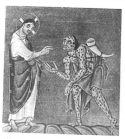

Hafensperren, Isolierungsplätzen, Quarantänen, Anzeigepflicht und Absonderung der Kranken und ihrer Pfleger, Desinfektion der Betten, Verbrennung alles nicht Abseifbaren aus der unmittelbaren Umgebung des Kranken oder Gestorbenen, schließlich Desinfektion der Waren, Geldstücke, Briefe im geschäftlichen Verkehr. Vollkommen durchschaut waren die Gefahren der Kontaktinfektion überhaupt und

Abb. 106. Aussätziger mit Horn (horngibruodr) um sich bemerklich zu machen, vor Christus. Deutsches Handschriftbild um 1000.

daraus die Sicherungsvorschriften erflossen, die dem 18. und 19. Jahrhundert prinzipiell kaum viel Neues zuzufügen übrig ließen. Und das alles in den ersten Jahrzehnten des 14. Jahrhunderts! Wie war diese große Wandlung zuwege gekommen? Sie geht in die Zeiten der verspotteten „Mönchsmedizin" zurück. Hier ist sogar direkt aus dem Boden der Priestermedizin Zukunftsreichstes erwachsen.

Die wohl schon in den Zeiten des klassischen Altertums sporadisch den atlantischen Küsten durch die Küstenschiffahrt in Spanien und Frankreich und weiter nördlich ausgesäte Lepra (und was man sonst darunter verstand) hatte im 5. und 6. Jahrhundert im Süden und Westen Frankreichs ihr Land hinein steigende Bedeutung gewonnen. Dem Episkopat stieß die Not der ihm anvertrauten Be-

völkerung ans Herz, und man besann sich auf die Priesterpflichten aus dem alten Bunde, die ja auch den Kirchenvätern des Ostens, allen voran Basileios dem Großen die Wege gewiesen hatten zu seinen klugen Absperrungshäusern für die Aussätzigen in Kaisareia usw. Das Konzil von Lyon vom Jahre 583 gibt Vorschriften gegen den freien Verkehr der Aussätzigen, die von weiteren Konzilien ausgebaut wurden. Das Edikt des Langobardenkönigs Rothari vom Jahre 644 verlangt die Isolierung der Leprösen. In wenigen Jahrhunderten wurde die Leprabekämpfung durch Vermeidung jeder Form von Kontakt und Ausatmungsübertragung aufs feinste ausgebaut bis zur Forderung besonderer Weihwasserbecken und Sitzplätze für die Aussätzigen in den Kirchen, solange man ihnen nicht besondere Kapellen zuwies. Besonders streng gehandhabt wurde die Vorschrift auch im Nahrungsmittelhandel. Die amtliche Schau für die Leprösen und ihre Beurteilung durch ärztliche Körperschaften war im 14. Jahrhundert bis in die feinsten Beurteilungsreglements ausgebaut. In Frankreich und Deutschland gab es gegen 10000 Isolierungshäuser

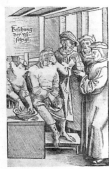

Abb. 107. Aussatzschau. Die Aerzte und Bader (den Blutkuchen auswaschend), 1517.

für Leprose ums Jahr 1400. Im zähen Kampfe hat man Fuß für Fuß der schleichenden Krankheit den Boden abgewonnen und sie schließlich zum Erlöschen gebracht. Aber schon hatte sich auch der Blick mächtig geweitet; der Begriff der „morbi contagiosi", der durch direkte Uebertragung ansteckenden Krankheiten, war den Aerzten des 13. Jahrhunderts allmählich in Fleisch und Blut übergegangen, unabhängig von der neuen Belehrung aus dem Osten. Erst 5, dann 8, dann 11, schließlich 13 ansteckende Krankheiten wurden aufgezählt. Zu Lepra, Influenza, Augenblennorrhoe und Trachom, Skabies, Impetigo kam bald Anthrax, Diphtherie, Erysipel, typhöse Fieber, Pest, sogar Lungenphthise usw. hinzu, die alle für an-

2 Images of leprosy, one from *c.* 1000 and one from *c.* 1500, from Theodor Meyer-Steineg and Karl Sudhoff, *Geschichte der Medizin im Überblick mit Abbildungen* (Jena, 1921).

Steineg, Professor of the History of Medicine at Jena, produced the first illustrated medical history (illus. 2).[59] They intended it to be a replacement for Schwalbe's outline history of medicine. This volume remained in print in updated form well into the 1960s.[60] In the introduction to the first edition they stressed the importance of the 208 images they reproduce as the central part of the innovations. They stressed further that these images are not *merely* illustrations but rather enhance the understanding of the material. Their images are all 'factual': portraits of the Great Men of medicine, of medical instruments, plates from Vesalius's anatomy and other technical manuals, as well as images of the patient in many contexts. Thus their use of images is absolutely indistinguishable from those undertaken in the late nineteenth century by ethnological museums collecting interesting objects from exotic cultures. One might add the illustrated book in high Modernism around the time of the Great War followed this tradition, when the 'Blue Riders' published their almanac of exotic objects from primitive cultures and Alfred Einstein published his collection of images of African art. The illustrated history became a repository for the historically exotic as well as the image of the 'Great Men' in the history of medicine.

Meyer-Steineg had used such visual material in his two books on ancient medicine.[61] The assumption behind all of these images is that contemporary photographs of ancient medical instruments have the same epistemological value as do portraits of Hippocrates or Malpighi. This was, for Meyer-Steineg, part of the underlying conception of the teaching of medicine as a link between past recovered and present experienced.[62]

The multiple, simultaneous meanings of these images are harnessed to the new professional role of the medical historian. Completely missing from this self-proclaimed first illustrated history of medicine are any references to mental illness, its treatment (with the exception of a portrait of Mesmer), and mental patients. Writing about medicine and its history – at least when illustrated – precluded dealing with the image of mental illness. The emphasis on the physical aspects of medicine in the age of the rise of psychosomatic medicine and psychoanalysis can only be understood as a conscious rejection of the premises of Charcot's popularizing attempt to use the illustration as a visual proof of his own theories of mental illness in a very different academic setting, the creation of modern clinical psychiatry. Indeed, by the time Sudhoff turned to formulating the basis for the history of medicine, Charcot's work (and his sense of his own visual antecedents) had fallen into scientific disrepute. Thus Sudhoff needed to segregate medical practice from medical history. History is a *Geisteswissenschaft* (the humanistic sciences), according to the philosopher Wilhelm Dilthey, and medicine, in terms of its nineteenth-century claims, is a *Naturwissenschaft* (the natural sciences). This distinction gives the same scholarly status associated with the natural sciences during this period to the humanities. It echoes in Haskell's definition cited above of the role of medical history. But this claim for parity between these two means of organizing knowledge gives equivalent value to two very different means of proof. It raises the role of 'interpretation' in the *Geisteswissenschaften* to the same level of the 'facts' in the *Naturwissenschaften*. Charcot elided these two means of proof, disguising his interpretation of history as 'facts' within the realm of the new specialty of psychiatry. In so doing he polluted the separation of a new, professional medical history from its professional roots in medical treatment. Sudhoff needed to separate these two models to establish himself as a historian. Interpreting images of madness would bring him (and Meyer-Steineg) back into the camp of Charcot, an approach that by the 1920s had totally fallen into disrepute, even in Paris.

The present volume addresses yet one other submerged question in the illustrated history of medicine that had been raised by Charcot. Charcot presumed a nation as his presumptive reader/viewer. In the 1880s it was necessary to address a more general audience of educated lay readers, such as Marcel Proust, and non-specialist physicians in the work that he and Richer published. Here it was important to create an image that linked Paris, as the putative cultural centre of Europe, with the image at the very centre of innovation in psychiatry. The view of the time was clearly that French clinical medicine was the best in the world, although German basic medical science was seen as slightly better than the French.[63] This was linked to notions of the modernization of techniques of analysis, such as the application of photography to the study of the mentally ill. If French science was only slightly more modern than German science, French visual culture was understood throughout Europe as inherently superior. French academic art of the time was in no way to be challenged by its German equivalent, and certainly the Impressionists defined the visual avant-garde for the rest of Europe.

The readership of Sudhoff and Meyer-Steineg's illustrated history of medicine, in which the history of 'French' psychiatry is missing except for a gesture toward its quack background through the image of Mesmer, clearly was expected to favour German historical science over that of the French. Sudhoff and Meyer-Steineg addressed the same audience as Charcot, and their intent was just as national. The audience was national (German) as well as international (scientific). The intent of their medical history was to 'give to German doctors and German medical science the world reputation it deserves' (p. 5). After the defeat of Germany in 1919 at the hands of, among others, the French, German science (especially historical science) had to be rescued from the charges of inferiority and partiality, especially in the light of the charges that German science was one of the tools of German imperial aggression. And the 'innovation' of the illustrated medical history, with its claim on the epistemology of nineteenth-century historical science, was used to buttress this claim for the 'evident' scientific superiority of German natural science. The appeal was to the broadest audience of educated readers, the *Bildungsbürgertum* that Sudhoff had not understood as his audience prior to the Great War.

The reason that Sudhoff could not lay claim to the arena of the illustrated medical history before 1920 was that this arena was already occupied in Germany. Even though Sudhoff and Meyer-Steineg's volume is the first self-proclaimed illustrated history of medicine, this was their own understanding of their project. Popular 'cultural' histories using medical imagery existed prior to their medical history. Hermann Peter's illustrated history of doctors and medicine with 153 images appeared in 1900 in a series on German cultural history.[64] Focusing on the period from 1500 to 1700, Peters does discuss and present the history of mental illness in his popular account of the 'progress' of medicine. More importantly, Eugen Holländer (1867–1932) had produced a series of illustrated 'histories' of medicine as reflected in the various visual sources mined by many 'serious' scholars, such as Meyer-Steineg and Sudhoff.[65] A number of the plates in Sudhoff and Meyer-Steineg's illustrated history came from Holländer. Sudhoff's professional opinion was that they were interesting sources of images but provided no professional insight into the world of medicine in which these images might have been used.[66]

Holländer was one of the first modern cosmetic surgeons in the 1890s. His medical interest in reconstituting the body aesthetically and his popular interest in how the body was represented in the world of visual culture were reflected in a number of historical studies beginning before the Great War. Holländer's work was hugely popular. His 'coffee-table' books were often reprinted. His audience was clearly the educated lay public as much as it was physicians. And he saw himself as the natural successor to Charcot and the School of Paris in terms of his interest in visual representations.[67] Thus the representations of mental illness play as great a role in Holländer's works as they did in those of Charcot and Richer. In the second edition of his history of medical caricature (1921), which appeared roughly at the same time as Meyer-Steineg and Sudhoff's first illustrated history of medicine, one can see a different use of images as the basis for analysis. First, like Meyer-Steineg and Sudhoff, Holländer uses the images to illustrate the progress of medicine. Unlike Meyer-Steineg and Sudhoff, Holländer's reliance on caricatures would tend to stress the 'unreal' qualities of the images. Yet in his chapter on 'mental illness' it is clear that the progressive tone of the volume is identical to that of Meyer-Steineg and Sudhoff. His text commands: Look how primitive the understanding of this illness was in early days. And his images repeat this theme. Thus he juxtaposes (pp. 198–9) a contemporaneous photograph from the Medical–Historical Museum in Amsterdam of eighteenth-century means of treatment with an early modern Dutch broadside on cutting the 'fool's stone' (illus. 3). He thus implies a visual link between the caricature of the fool and the world of the treatment of

fie Anteil an der Spezies – Menſch – als durch Stimme und Geſtalt, und alles andere ſei viel weniger als Vieh (Entwurf zu ſeiner Anatomie).

Dieſer ganz Dummen nahmen ſich nun mit Vorliebe die herumfahrenden Gaukler und Scharlatane an. Die alten Hippokratiſchen Vorſchriften gegen die Epilepſie, am Kopf das Glüheiſen anzuleßen oder die Stirnvene zu ſchröpfen – Aretäus empfiehlt ſogar die Trepanation –, kamen wieder zu Ehren und wurden, wie alle modernen Mittel, über-

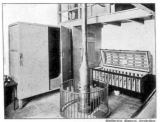

Fig. 97. Rollkutſche und Krampfbett.

trieben. Es bildeten ſich die Steinſchneideſpezialiſten, die bei Kopfkrämpfen und allerlei nervöſen Zuſtänden angeblich Steine aus dem Kopfe ſchnitten. In der »Medizin in der klaſſiſchen Malerei« haben wir dies Kapitel bereits behandelt und gezeigt, wie Jan Steen dieſem Thema ſchon allen Wiß und kauſtiſchen Humor vorweg genommen hat. Streiften dieſe gemalten Satiren gegen die menſchliche Dummheit bereits auf das karikaturiſtiſche Gebiet über, ſo gab der Gegenſtand auch noch Veranlaſſung zu den erſten wirklichen Karikaturen dieſer Art. Henri Meige, der verdienſtvolle und zielbewußte Hüter des Charcotſchen Erbes in Frankreich, hat in einer intereſſanten Monographie in der Iconographie de la Salpêtrière bereits die betreffenden Blätter veröffentlicht, die teil-

weiſe große Raritäten geworden ſind. Das Bekannteſte iſt ein von Allardt geſchnittenes Blatt, welches dadurch beſonders in weiteſte Kreiſe drang,

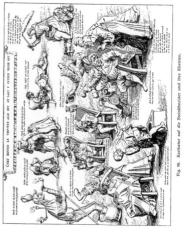

daß die Zeichnungen und Stöcke deſſelben durch die Veränderung der Inſchriften zu einer Verhöhnung des berühmten Kolonialaktienſchwindels benüßt wurden. Das Originalblatt trägt die Überſchrift: Comt Mannen en Vrouwen alle bey – en laet v ſnyden vande key.

---

3 Photograph of a museum with a vertigo-inducing machine and other apparatus for the treatment of the mentally ill; and an early modern broadside on the 'cutting of the fool's stone', from Eugen Holländer, *Die Karikatur und Satire in der Medizin, Medikokunsthistorische Studie* (2nd edition, Stuttgart, 1921). Madness was imagined as localized in the head of the mad person much like the myth of the jewel in the head of the toad; remove the offending 'stone of madness' and the madness was cured.

the mentally ill. But more importantly, he assumed that a contemporary photograph of a museum exhibit would be the equivalent of his own project: creating a visual museum of the antiquarian fantasies about mental illness and its treatment in the past. When Holländer evokes contemporary treatment of illness in his volume, he is much more reticent about drawing the modalities of treatment into question. His final chapter on contemporary medical caricatures stresses the altered social role of the physician, the physician's claim to high social status, not his ability to cure. (Given the contemporary anxiety about female physicians, this is even the case in one of the caricatures aimed against female physicians.) Using caricatures gave Holländer a substantial advantage over more 'serious' historians of the medical image of the nineteenth century, such as Choulant, as they provide access to cultural attitudes toward medicine, and that is indeed what he examines. This approach is clearly rejected by Sudhoff, who needs to seek selected facts to explain contemporary realities of medical practice. Attitude is simply too subjective an aspect of images to concern 'serious' historians of medicine such as Sudhoff.

Here the status of the image in the historiography of psychiatry can be stressed. All of the uses point towards their truthfulness, yet each 'truth' is developed in terms of its ability to create a professional identity. To cite Michel Foucault in this context, 'a proposition must fulfill complex and heavy requirements to be able to belong to the grouping of a discipline; before it can be called true or false, it must be "in the true"'. And why is it important to belong to a discipline? To gain the power of being 'called true or false'.[68] Images, at least in early medical historiography, were the field for conflicts over professionalization and national identity. Images placed the author in a specific relationship to the reader and to the reader's presumed use of such images for enjoyment as well as education. (Meyer-Steineg and Sudhoff stress in their introduction the Enlightenment appropriation of Horace's ideal of education *and* amusement.)

But I would add that the actual power of the visual image made it the natural space for such debates. For the historical image, especially the image of the mentally ill and those who treat mental illness, evokes a specific type of anxiety about location and identification. Each image provides simultaneous, multiple meanings that the viewer accesses immediately and attempts to reduce to a coherent, single meaning. Some of these meanings are found within the image itself. In a reading of an image the observer can find either an accurate interpretation of the image (an interpretation buttressed by documentation of parallel discourses from the time) or a false reading (a reading through the history of misreadings of an image over the course of its reception). But some of these meanings are embedded in the historian's ability to shape and delimit the function of the use of images because of the self-definition of the historian's agenda. Such suppressed readings come to be part of the history of missing readings that shape our present understanding of the image. They are the 'secrets and non-interchangeable roles' that Foucault sees even in 'discourse that is published and free from all ritual' (p. 122). The rarity of the images of the mentally ill in the scholarly work on the history of psychiatry stems from such a repressed secret.

In *Disease and Representation* (1988) I stressed the representation of illness as the stage on which the cultural fantasies of every member of society – physician and lay alike – could be played out. Such images are found in a free space, within which parallel discourses are developed to exploit the ambiguity of the image. The now limited and interpreted image is itself a place in which there is a shared idea of healing and illness, and that idea is reified by the image. But, of course, such a view assumes that the multiple, simultaneous meanings of the image, meanings that provide an inherent ambiguity to each and every image, are vitiated rather than repressed. What is undertaken is a communal or individual repression of the ambiguity of the image itself. The anxieties about illness are replaced by control over the image. As we shall see in this study, the images can seem to be controlled, while the 'illnesses' constructed seem always to be beyond control. This anxiety is played out in the world of representations for historians and for readers, as it is a safer and more controlled world than the world of illness, real or imagined. To do so it is necessary to control the multiple, simultaneous meanings of visual representations and to focus on a seemingly concrete, single interpretation. This book will attempt to open up a set of images that represent health and illness and show how the problem of simultaneity complicates the interpretation of such images.

2 Again Madness as a Test Case: The Psychiatric Image and Multiple, Simultaneous Meanings

To examine the potential of the simultaneous, multiple, and often contradictory meanings inherent in all images let me turn to a series of representations of mental illness. My examples are, for the most part, relatively little known but they span images of the mentally ill from the traditions of medical illustration to high and popular art from the past two centuries. All of these images could be used in all four of the ways outlined in the opening section of this book. I have chosen the representation of 'madness' and the 'insane' as one further corrective to the difficulties that scholars in the history of medicine have had in using precisely such images. These images 'control' a double anxiety. First, they bound the general anxiety about madness and instability that we all share, and second, they reduce the parallel anxiety about the multiple meanings of the images themselves to a controlled, single interpretation. This double anxiety about mental and interpretative destabilization is linked in the observation of such images.

The control evidenced in these images thus provides a pleasure on the illustrated page, even when the image itself is neither 'beautiful' nor 'pleasant'. We share the sense that Alice had, sitting in the warm sun, watching her sister read some heavy tome, that 'what is the use of a book without pictures or conversations?' But the pleasure is also that of having repressed anxiety. The presuppositions about the nature of mental illness inscribed make these images real: they provide access to some level of experienced reality. Each of these images employ specific aesthetic techniques to achieve its ends, techniques that are so accepted in Western visual culture as to seem 'natural'. Additionally these pictures provide access to the perpetuation of a fantasy of 'beauty and health' and 'ugliness and illness'. The tension between these two moments places viewers always in the role of the distanced observer, no matter what the reality of their health. This is the least complex level of the image's multiple, simultaneous meanings. For the aesthetics of the body that associates the 'beautiful' with the 'healthy' confuses two spheres of experience in a direct and insistent manner. Thus these

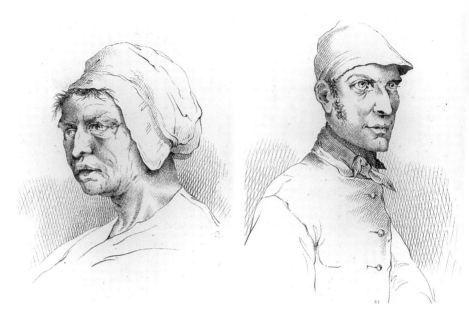

images provide a means of dealing with the anxieties about the illnesses represented. For the images themselves become the space in which the anxieties are controlled. Their finitude, their boundedness, their inherent limitation provide a distance analogous to the distance the observer desires from the 'reality' of the illness portrayed. For here we can 'see' and 'sense' the abyss between the 'healthy' and the 'ill'.

Let us begin at the highest level of medical science at the very beginning of the nineteenth century. Joseph Guislain (1797–1860) was Professor of Medicine at Ghent and the most important Belgian alienist of his time as well as the reformer of the Belgian asylum system. His influence was felt across Europe. In his standard handbook of lectures on insanity written in the 1820s, he provided a micro-catalogue of three images of three asylum patients to illustrate three states of mental illness: a patient suffering from maniacal melancholy (illus. 4), an ecstatic patient (illus. 5), and an idiot (illus. 6). These three categories encapsulate his nosological system, the system by which he organized his categories of mental illness.[1] The portraits served as illustrations for his published lectures. They substituted for the 'real' patients to which medical students could have access only with difficulty in the reformed asylum that Guislain advocated. Thus the very notion of an 'illustration' in Guislain's work has a relationship to his conception of the very definition of mental illness as well as the appropriate treatment of the mentally ill. The introduction of images within medical textbooks dealing with the mentally ill are part of the

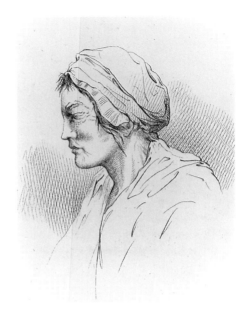

4 'A woman with maniacal melancholy', from Joseph Guislain's *Vorträge über Geistes-Krankheiten*, trans. Heinrich Laehr (Berlin, 1854).

5 'An ecstatic patient', from Guislain's *Vorträge über Geistes-Krankheiten*.

6 'An idiot, from Guislain's *Vorträge über Geistes-Krankheiten*.

asylum reform movement, as they provide a substitute for 'real' patients.

In the world of eighteenth-century representations of madness or the insane there was always a catalogue of the range of insanity available to the artist and the viewer. It was necessary to be able to distinguish between the mad and the sane. The assumption was that the sane observer/artist knew who were mad because they were located in spaces labelled as 'madhouses'. Thus images in the eighteenth century – images in a world that had begun to question the meaning of the traditional ascription and, perhaps, even of definitions of madness – were always cast in a way so as to localize the insane. The world of Guislain is very different. For him the trick was to teach those who had to deal with the mad how to differentiate between the mad and the sane, if the normative definitions no longer held. The observer could not simply assume that societal signs provided sufficient information; rather, that only professional (medical) training enabled the physician/observer to learn to see the insane in a world in which insanity was not always overtly marked. These covert signs could be taught, but they were not self-evident.

But how does Guislain represent his trio of patients? Do they look different, from, let us say, an idealized portrait of the alienist of the time, the sort of portrait that historians of psychiatry might use to illustrate their histories of the Great Men of psychiatry? These portraits follow the aesthetic conventions for images reproducible in medical textbooks during the first half of the nineteenth century. Lithographs and engravings had their own aesthetic code through which they communicated certain 'realities'. Thus the 'melancholic' patient is visually marked by the blackness of her skin, which traditionally signalled the presence of melancholy ('black bile'). The greater darkness of the portrait's visage is created through cross-hatching. Such aesthetic conventions are standard to all multiple images created in Western art at the time. They are aesthetic responses to illnesses and present these illnesses within the constraints of image-making. Within the world of medical imagery, they are also images of the ill and are therefore, as we shall discuss in the next chapter, evocations of the ugly. In most somatic illnesses such a link can rely on physical signs; in the representation of mental illness, 'ugliness' is a symbolic reflection of the imagined inner state of the patient. Here the externalization of the perceived inner world of the patient presents the fantasy of the physician and artist about the meaning of the patient's appearance.

Thus these portraits stand in a specific tradition within the psychiatric literature of their day. They are similar to many of the standard images of the mentally ill in the atlases of the first half of the nineteenth century. They provided half-portraits with the emphasis on the face and the physiognomy to reveal to the trainee the illness that was written on the face. It is the face that was central to all analysis, for traditionally it is the visage that is supposed to provide access to the character of the individual observed. The medical training of young physicians, moreover, was always in aesthetic terms, and this is further inscribed in Guislain's portraits. All of these portraits are 'ugly', in implied reference to the implied standard that the healthy is the beautiful, and they are 'uglier' the more severe was their illness. The visible gestures toward the invisible. Here there is the echo of the model of classical aesthetics employed by Philippe Pinel in the very first textbook of psychiatry.[2] And all of this is encapsulated in the manner by which Guislain represents the patient's manner of seeing the world through his image of their gaze.

In a world in which learning (that is, the rational) is to be undertaken through training the medical student's sight, it is of little wonder that the very gaze of the patient comes to be the measure of the intensity of the illness and the ability of the physician to cure. The most severely ill of the three is the third. Blind, her physiognomy is as blank as her future. The introspective gaze of the melancholic marks her impairment. Her inability to look directly at the observer is not merely an accident of placement, but a comment on her diagnosis and prognosis. The image of the ecstatic incorporates all of the anti-religious feeling of these early reformers. Religious ecstasy is seen as a psychopathological state, and any form of mental illness that can be understood in terms of such a model must be deep-seated if not permanent. His gaze, marked by bulging eyes, seems to see beyond the observer. Treatment as well as diagnosis was rooted in such a physiognomic analysis. This reduction of the patient to an aesthetic abstraction is, as Richard Gray has commented, in line with the physiognomist's need to understand all autonomous bourgeois subjects as aesthetic constructions.[3] Aesthetics was thus rooted in the equation of 'beauty/health' and 'ugliness/illness'.

Yet there is also a second set of hidden implications in Guislain's seemingly self-evident equation of physiognomic ugliness and mental impairment. Here a second visual source from the 1850s can be of help. August Krauss, in his study of how to make sense out of madness (1859), provided a table of animal analogies to forms of mental impairment of a type well known as early as the Renaissance (illus. 7).[4]

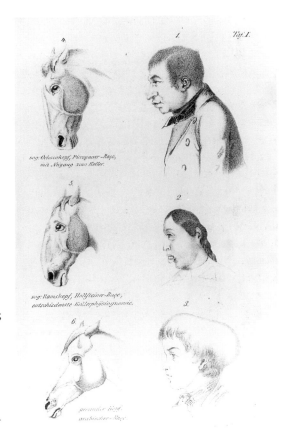

7 Analogies of various forms of madness to the various breeds of horse (top and bottom: 'ox-head', Pinzgauer stock, tendency to rage; 'ram's-head', Hollsteiner stock, choleric physiognomy; heathy head, Arabian stock); from August Krauss's 'Der Sinn in Wahnsinn' in *Allgemeine Zeitschrift für Psychiatrie* XVII (1859).

Here an additional question, unstated yet implied by Guislain, is introduced: How much does the mental state of the individuals depicted relate to the social groups in which they function? For it is evident that the construction of categories of 'beauty/health' and 'ugliness/illness' relate to the aesthetics of the group or class as well as to individual aesthetics. Here Krauss's introduction of the question of 'race', i.e., the physiognomy and character of various breeds of horse, can be seen to be encoded in the high science of his day. 'Character' and 'race' become linked in the world of animal analogies. For the eighteenth-century physiognomists, such as J. K. Lavater, categories such as race were assumed to have physiognomic, and therefore characterological, validity.

The physician is trained to see the individual as a representative of the nosological category of mental illness, a category that is as unwavering and as 'real' as breeds of horse. In both cases the reality can be measured by the appearance of the individual's physiognomy. Here again it is the idiot whose permanent incapacity is the model for the most impaired and the ugliest on Krauss's scale of seeing the insane. Again it is the gaze represented by the image of the eyes that is the index of difference. All of Krauss's analogies are encoded already in Guislain's visual scale of impairment. Indeed, even in Guislain's implied nosology there is an inherent hierarchy of impairment because of the historical relationship between 'beauty/health' and 'ugliness/ illness'. Thus 'race', in Krauss's sense referring only to breeds of horse, becomes part of the discourse of seeing the insane; the categories of medical and psychiatric nosology come to be categories of organization like the breeds of horse.

The 'normal/beautiful' individual (in reality, the physician as the idealized observer) is missing in this model of seeing the insane. The aesthetic hierarchy runs from the least impaired (the least ugly individual) to the ugliest (most impaired), and is linked through the very act of seeing because of the prestige of sight, the most 'rational' of senses, after the Enlightenment.[5] If we accept that the gaze of the physician represents 'health' and 'beauty' and that of the patient 'illness' and 'ugliness', we can observe their implied juxtaposition even in the ironic image of the hypnotist (or mesmerist, the eighteenth-century term) and his patient (illus. 8) made in 1826 by Louis Boilly (1761–1845). Here the closed eyes of the old and grizzled female patient mask her gaze and represent the therapeutic trance with its potentially exploitative functions. The young and handsome hypnotist does not represent the 'good' physician even though he shares some of the 'good' physician's attributes. For by the 1820s in France, mesmer-

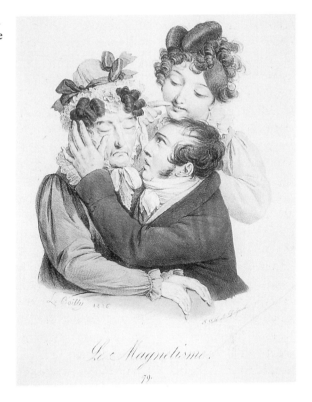

8 *Mesmerism*, Louis Boilly's image of the mesmerist and his patients, 1826.

ism was understood as a form of charlatanism. The staring eyes of the mesmerist, like those of the ecstatic patient in Guislain's text, point toward the religious analogy. Here the quack is as 'mad' as the patient. The contrastive figure of the next patient, the beautiful young woman, provides a commentary on the falsity of the hypnotist, who will treat even those who are clearly not in need of treatment.

Guislain's and Krauss's images fulfil all the categories of images that have been used in the history of psychiatry: they are 'illustrations', they provided access for medical students and physicians to 'real' patients through their case material, they employed very specific aesthetic techniques and theories of medical portraiture, and they provide insight into the fantasies of the meaning ascribed to the mind and the body in the first half of the nineteenth century. Boilly's image is a satire on a fashionable, false madness and its equally false treatment. The caricature of the mentally ill, parallel to the medical illustration of the insane, emphasizes the aesthetic qualities ascribed to the representation as well as to the disease process. For the insane are not only unaesthetic in their appearance, they have lost the ability to discriminate aesthetically. The inability to distinguish between the beautiful and

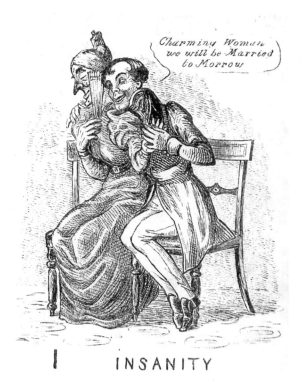

Charming Woman we will be Married to Morrow

I INSANITY

the ugly as objects of attraction is a clear indicator of madness in popular representations of the insane, of their insanity. Love madness, a nosological category for physicians dealing with mental illness from the time of J.E.D. Esquirol in the 1830s, destroys all ability to distinguish between aesthetic qualities. Thus when we move from 'medical' illustrations made for the training or edification of physicians to 'popular' images, the dimension open only to the professional's gaze becomes an overt or public statement available to all viewers.

The caricature from 1837 of insanity as love madness by the British artist C. J. Grant (illus. 9) depicts this as well as implies the economic imperative for younger men to marry older, wealthy women. This image is part of an alphabet in which each of the plates represents a medical specialty or illness. Insanity, in the abstract, is represented by 'love madness'. It is society that makes such creatures mad by defying the 'natural' aesthetic categories. Each – the 'ugly/old' woman and the 'beautiful/young' man – is mad. The historical trope is an ancient one, the marriage of 'May' and 'December', but the gender roles are reversed. In Chaucer or in the theme of the mad Aristotle it is the old man who pursues the young bride, to his detriment. Here it is the economic pursuit of the old woman by the young man that marks both as mad. To make their madness obvious to the viewer, Grant uses the typical exaggeration of features that is found in the work of eighteenth-century caricaturists such as Hogarth or Rowlandson. Here the pock-marked, darkened face of the woman, with its prominent, hooked nose, and the inappropriate grin on the face of her foppish suitor, points to their bad character: false modesty on her part; greed on his. These caricatures use the same aesthetics of physiognomy and the juxta-position of 'beauty/health' and 'ugliness/illness' that structure the medical images. The juxtaposition of action and appearance provides a further clue, for the young man is only to be seen as 'insane' in the context of his suit. His false exterior ('beauty') is itself revealed to be a sign of his mental illness. The decline of Hogarth's Tom Rakewell – from his healthy life in the country through his capitulation to the seductions of London to his eventual incarceration in Bedlam (illus. 10) – is figured in his physical decline. And his foppishness is part of that decline even though it does not appear to be so until we have seen the entire sequence of images. Grant's gesture toward his type of Hogarthian rejection of a false male beauty is both a sign of a popular awareness of the aesthetics of 'beauty/health' and 'ugliness/illness' but also an intertextual reference that would have been evident to any British reader.

The images of 'health' and 'illness' thus employ a level of artistic intertextuality that is vital to any understanding of their impact. Art quotes art. A radical reorganization of the aesthetics of the normal can be captured in George Bellows's version of the ball of the insane, his lithograph *Dance in a Madhouse* (illus. 11). This essentially Late Victorian image has a long history (one that I traced back to the Middle Ages in my *Seeing the Insane*). As in all of these evocations of the 'mad ball' in the nineteenth and early twentieth centuries, Bellows's lithograph adds the wild and uncontrolled movement attributed to the insane to the physiognomy and physical positions traditionally associ-ated with the mentally ill in Western art. The grotesque physiognomy of the inmates points toward the aesthetics of madness found in Grant and Boilly. But it is also the classically melancholic and passive position of the inmates on the benches as well as the oddly matched dancing couples, that provided Bellows with this image of the asylum as microcosm of the world.[6]

The asylum as the microcosm of the world is a well-worn visual theme in representations of the world of the mentally ill. The asylum as a device for social comment requires that the inmates possess a particular and identifiable physiognomy and posture, as the physical

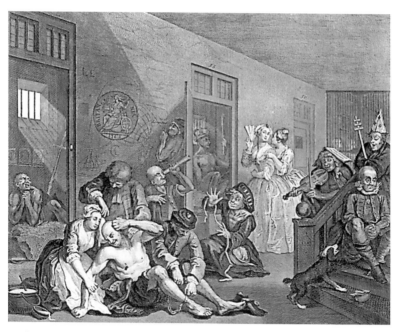

10 The final plate of William Hogarth's *A Rake's Progress*, 1735.

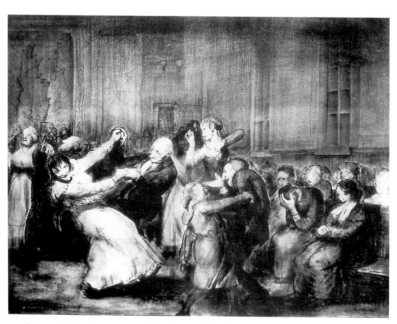

11 George Bellows's version of the image of the ball of the insane in his lithograph *Dance in a Madhouse*, 1917.

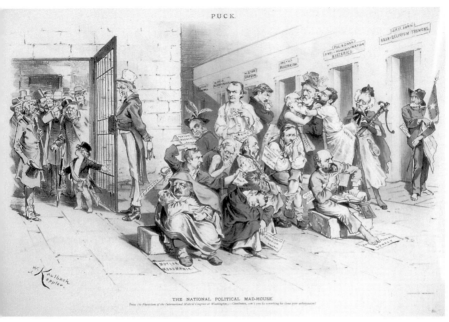

12　*The National Political Mad-House*: Joseph Keppler's image of the world of American politics as an asylum, in an 1887 issue of the American magazine *Puck*.

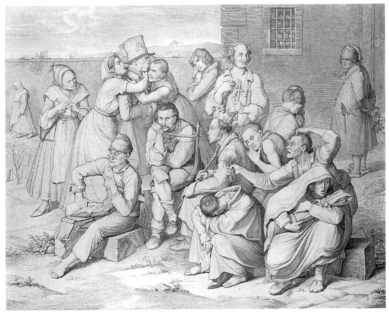

13　Engraving by C. H. Merz, after Wilhelm Kaulbach, *Madhouse*, 1835.

body of the mentally ill makes the 'perverse' or 'degenerate' character of the inmates visible. In an 1887 caricature from the American humour magazine *Puck* (1877–1918), all of American Reconstruction politics is to be found in the madhouse (illus. 12). It was drawn by the famed lithographer Joseph Keppler, who was born in Vienna in 1838, went to America in 1868 (and to New York in 1873) and died in 1894. From the 'monomaniacal' Benjamin 'Silver Spoons' Butler of Massachusetts, running for President on the Greenback Party, to the young William Jennings Bryan and his 'new crusade', to Charles A. Dana of the *New York Sun* as a feminized hysteric, to Henry George, his 'anti-property lunacy' represented by a copy of his *Progress and Property* opened on his lap – every kind of American politics is on display in this asylum. The physicians attending a medical convention in Washington look in through the open door as Puck asks: 'Can't you do something for these poor unfortunates?' This is a heavily, perhaps even crudely, political reworking of an earlier set of images.

What is striking about Keppler's image is that it is a figure-by-figure redoing of the two most influential asylum scenes of the nineteenth century, Wilhelm Kaulbach's *Madhouse* (illus. 13) of 1835 and the final print of Hogarth's *A Rake's Progress* of a century earlier (illus. 10). The central group of figures is to be found in Kaulbach (this reference is actually given in the image), although the setting is not the open yard of Kaulbach's engravings but the closed ward of Hogarth's Bedlam. Kaulbach's image is selfconsciously archaic, reflecting as much a German reading of Hogarth as the real experience of an unreformed German asylum to which Kaulbach was exposed as a young man. Indeed, the open 'cells' in the *Puck* image echo the cells in Hogarth's asylum with their political reference to 'mad' kings. And the figures of Puck and the physicians serve the same role as the visitors in Hogarth's world – to observe and be commented on by the viewer of the print, who stands outside the world of the inhabitant as well as outside the world of the visitor. Here we can see the shift from the eighteenth-century experience with the mentally ill to the world of the image in and from the reformed asylum, with its distance from daily experience and its need to train the clinician's gaze. For the political caricature, the Hogarthian model of the asylum as the microcosm of the world needed to be evoked. Here the question is one of ironic 'tone'. The artist must be sure that the observer can immediately see the world of politics as the world of the mad. No ambiguity is permitted in political evocations such as this.

The intertextual citation of these two images hardly evokes the aesthetic world of the asylum any more than any 'real' picture of a late nineteenth-century Washington asylum, such as St Elizabeth's. Each political figure becomes the equivalent of a figure in these earlier images of the asylum, and the viewer, well trained to read these images in terms of their physiognomy and character, can understand the madness of the political world. Yet neither Hogarth nor Kaulbach seem to invite this interpretation. Is it simply that Keppler could evoke the madhouse with bits and pieces from Hogarth and Kaulbach to generate a composite madhouse with its prototypal inhabitants? Or does he pick up on a theme hidden well within these prototypes – the political world as the asylum? In Hogarth this theme is clear. In the cell labelled '55' in his image (mirrored in the cells at the rear of the image from *Puck*) there sits a man gone mad with pride, wearing a straw crown and holding a broken stick as a sceptre. He is observed by the visitors as he urinates. Next to his cell Britannia is drawn on the wall; her loose hair represents the madness of the state. Politics are inscribed heavily in Hogarth's madhouse. Kaulbach 'quotes' Hogarth by introducing the mad king into the central position in his image. His mock crown and stick-sceptre reflect the political world gone mad. The reality of politics in the macro-asylum of the world is mirrored in political figures within the world of madness. Thus the image in *Puck* is indeed intertextual in its direct use of political themes and its expansion to include all the figures of this new macro-Bedlam, Washington.

In the world of nineteenth-century caricature, the frame comprises the earlier images that relate to antiquated, though culturally powerful, notions of madness. Thus reality is the world of the artistic image of high art to which the caricature makes reference. The fantasies are those about the world of politics rather than the world of madness, and the intertextual gesture relates the images drawn from the world of high art through the iconography of madness to the world of politics. The artist is quite comfortable when eliding these two images, neither one of which has any relationship to the daily reality of madness in the 1880s. But all relate through ideas of the aesthetic and its relationship to the moral and the beautiful.

The manipulation and alteration of images is not limited to the drawings and caricatures that represented the idea of mental illness during the late nineteenth and early twentieth centuries. Photographs, too, followed the juxtaposition of ideas of 'beauty/health' and 'ugliness/illness' in their representation of the mentally ill. Joseph Parrish (1818–91), editor of the *American Psychological Journal* in 1883–4, took photographs for an album at the Imbecile Asylum at Burlington, New Jersey, in 1886. These images are all like those used in the first American book illustrated with actual photographs of the mentally ill,

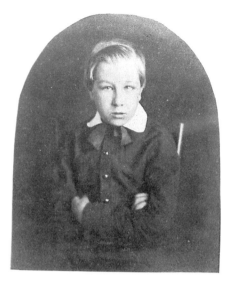

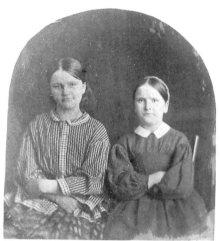

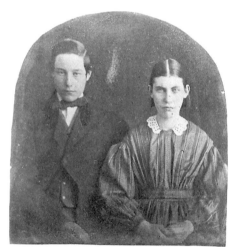

14, 15, 16 Photographs of inmates of the Imbecile Asylum in Burlington, New Jersey, assembled by Joseph Parrish, 1886.

published by Parrish's friend, Isaac Kerlin (1858–93), the superintendent of the Pennsylvania Institute for Feeble Minded Children in Elwyn.[7] Idiocy, as we have seen, provided the ultimate test for the relationship between the physiognomy of the insane and the ability to create visible nosological categories for mental illness and deficiency. Some of Parrish's images, like those used by Kerlin, are portraits in which the impairment seemed to be 'invisible'; others, where there is some physiological anomaly, posed the inmate in a manner so as to stress the visual difference of the mentally ill (illus. 14–16). Such images had a practical function – to provide source material for institutional fundraising. The two types of images stressed the poten-

17 A 'wanted poster' in a supplement to a 1905 issue of the German magazine *Psychiatrische-Neurologische Wochenschrift*, asking for the identification of the person pictured.

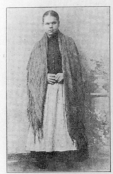

Beiblatt zu Nr. 32 der Psychiatr.-Neurolog. Wochenschrift.

4. November 1905.

Verlag von Carl Marhold, Halle a. S.

Liste zu ermittelnder unbekannter Geisteskranker.
Nr. 34.

Am 20. April 1904, abends 9¹/₂ Uhr, wurde die nebenstehend abgebildete Frauensperson in Siemianowitz, Kreis Kattowitz, obdachlos und umherirrend aufgegriffen und nach Feststellung ihrer Geistesschwäche dem dortigen Hedwigsstift zugeführt, später der Prov.-Heil- und Pflegeanstalt zu Lublinitz überwiesen.

Ausser dem Namen „Marenka" vermag die sehr schwerhörige und hochgradig stammelnde, polnische, ca. 25 Jahre alte Idiotin nichts über ihre Person anzugeben. Sie ist 156 cm gross, untersetzt, hat dunkelblonde Haare und Augenbrauen, braune Augen, leicht eingesunkenen Nasenrücken, verdickten Nasenknorpel, Nasenpolypen, schniefende Athmung bei verschlossenem Munde, dicke Lippen und mässig grosse Kropfgeschwulst. Zähne in gutem Zustande. Geht etwas schleppend und nach vorn geneigt. Plattfüsse. — Kleidung: Dunkelgrau karrirtes Umschlagetuch, blau und weissgeblumte Kattunjacke, blaue Leinwandschürze, schwarzer wollartiger Rock mit roter handbreiter Einfassung, grauer Leinwandunterrock, schwarze Tuchschuhe mit Ledereinfassung. Sie trug in der Hand einen zusammengelegten weissgeblumten Kattunrock.

Angaben, welche zur Ermittelung der Herkunft dieser Person dienen können, wolle man unter IIa 14956 dem Herrn Landeshauptmann von Schlesien mittheilen.

tial socialization of the inmates in the asylum setting as well as their impairment.

Another function that some of these images had was to contribute to the day-to-day reality of record-keeping. Thus many of the Continental journals of psychiatry aimed at asylum directors and physicians were accompanied by loose sheets (illus. 17). Unlike Parrish's images in Kerlin, a caption is needed to frame each one, for the asylum directors would need to know all that could be known about, say, this unknown person of 1905 if they should recognize her as an escapee or a former inmate. The frame, as necessary in this most pragmatic of images as the image itself, shorn of its aesthetic quality and stripped down to a Bertillon image for identification, needs to be contextualized. The fantasies of difference in Parrish's photographs are suspended. Here is an unknown, unnamed individual, who cannot herself tell who she is. It is not her gaze or her physiognomy or her position that marks her impairment, but the frame of the asylum director's caption, seeking her identity. Here the movement is *from* the photograph, hopefully to evoke an informed response on the part of a specific viewer. The question of the audience of the image thus becomes a factor in using it in writing the history of mental illness. It is with the audience that there lies a qualitative difference between Parrish's image and this wanted poster. Yet one can argue that the viewer of 1905 could easily distinguish the type of 'reality' that these photographs represented. Each photograph represents in its own way a means of capturing the nature of mental illness as defined by the functional use of the photograph within the asylum setting.

The nineteenth-century photograph gives us a sense of the 'realities' of life in the asylum, but the qualities ascribed to these realities are to no little degree effects of the photographic techniques of that day. The difference between the New Jersey and German photographs from late twentieth-century ones is sufficient to distort the difference between these two images. Our sense of what is aesthetically 'normal' in photographs is sufficiently different from the seemingly antiquated image by Parrish and the one in the wanted poster to make both seem to function for us in a similar manner. We must disentangle the multiple, simultaneous meanings inscribed in both in order to differentiate one from the other.

The shift between means of representing 'beauty/health' and 'ugliness/illness' through photographs of the mentally ill can be judged best once a new variable is introduced. Let us take two images that had a 'real' physiognomic intent, i.e., were part of atlases of medical physiognomy and were understood as presenting classic cases of mental illnesses in the late nineteenth and early twentieth centuries. For medical physiognomy is not 'merely' the subjective impression of physicians, but a diagnostic science. The physician's analysis of signs and symptoms on the face is part of the classical repertory of diagnosis from the Greeks to the present. No clearer set of contrasts could be found than two images of Graves's Disease, the first from Byrom Bramwell's *Atlas of Clinical Medicine* of 1894 (illus. 18) and the second from Carl Fervers's physiognomy of illness of 1935 (illus. 19). Here the line between somatic and psychological definitions of 'mental illness' vanishes. For centuries the physical sign of the exophthalmic goitre was employed as a standard sign in reading the physiognomy of the insane.[8] In terms of nineteenth-century concepts of mental illness, Graves's Disease was thought to be neurological (i.e., somatic) in origin. Its signs and symptoms are goitre, cardiac arrhythmia, increased apprehensiveness and fear, eyelid retraction, and a compulsive stare. Although there is a clinical difference between endemic goitre, usually the result of iodine insufficiency, and Graves's Disease, the external signs and symptoms (except for cretinism) overlap. The overlapping of these two somatic syndromes with their symptom of mental retardation

48

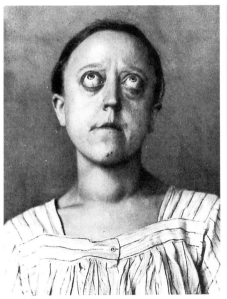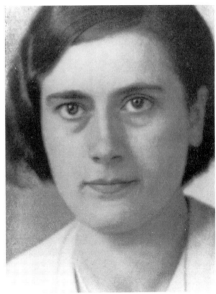

18 The physiognomy of a woman suffering from Graves's Disease, from Byrom Bramwell's *Atlas of Clinical Medicine* (Edinburgh, 1894).

19 The physiognomy of a woman suffering from Graves's Disease, from Carl Fervers's *Der Ausdruck des Kranken* (Munich, 1935).

or confusion led to their conflation as a category of mental illness. Graves's Disease is found most frequently in mature women and is caused by malfunction of the thyroid gland. Thus there is a clear gendering of the illness and an understanding that a goitre mars the aesthetic nature of the female patient. But more importantly, as Freud commented on a dead patient when confronted by her sister who too suffered from Graves's disease: 'The victims of Graves's disease, as has often been observed, have a marked facial resemblance to one another; and in this case this typical likeness was reinforced by a family one.'[9] Each sufferer of Graves's Disease looks like every other sufferer and the mental state of each is similar. Thus the diagnostic justification for an analysis of the relationship between the appearance of the patient and the patient's mental status.

From the 1890s to the 1930s the actual endocrinological basis of Graves's Disease was well known. By the 1880s the work of Felix Semon and Victor Horelsey and, after 1900, the work of David Marine, had documented the relationship between thyroid deficiency and the nervousness of Graves's Disease. But in the 1890s Byrom Bramwell provided an image that looked more exaggeratedly insane than does Fervers's representation from the mid-1930s. The subtle physiognomy of the somatic illness that needs interpretation replaces the overt and crass representation of the mentally ill. For Bramwell's image still needed to evoke the context of mental illness; Fervers's image no longer need to do this. Bramwell can use the actual symptom of the bulging eyes of the patient and, in finding a patient with an exaggerated version of this symptom, can stress the association with the older trope of the bulging, and therefore disrupted, gaze of the insane. Fervers finds a case in which this symptom is present, as it most certainly would be, but in an understated, subtle manner. That both are women points to the gendering of the illness itself. Yet Bramwell's image stresses the distortion and deformity resulting from the illness; Fervers's only hints at it.

By the 1930s Graves's Disease had moved out of the world of the physiognomy of the insane, a world evoked by Parrish's image and the wanted poster, to the world of somatic illness. To no little degree, this shift from the stigmatization of 'ugliness/illness' was the result of the ability to treat thyroid illnesses. With Emil Kocher's thyroidectomy, the work of George Murray on the use of the thyroids of sheep for the treatment of myxoedema, and Thomas Dunhill's surgical procedure for the removal of a exophthalmic goitre, the basis for considering the 'nervousness' or 'cretinism' of thyroid illnesses as forms of 'mental illness' was completely undermined. This can be 'seen' in these two images.

All representations in this exercise in reading the multiple, simultaneous images of 'beauty/health' and 'ugliness/illness' can be shown to have interlocking functions. They come from the medical literature (Guislain, Krauss, Bramwell, Fervers) as well as from high (Boilly, Bellows) and popular art (Grant, Keppler). All provide us with insights into some realities, whether social or physiological; all provide us with some insight into the fantasies about mental illness and its aesthetics; all use traditions and devices to refer to the world of aesthetic objects and their conventions. And all control the images and the range of interpretation, whether those limits are contextualized in the discussion of the images or present in the very structure of the image itself. Yet each representation provides the viewer with multiple, simultaneous meanings that need to be controlled just as much as does the anxiety about identifying oneself with the image of the mad. As we picture health and illness, we bring to the images an entire arsenal of aesthetic associations, and we see the world in terms of beauty and ugliness. These associations provide a means of placing ourselves as observers not only of these images but of our own bodies, bodies inherently in danger of illness.

3 The Ugly and the Beautiful: Cross-Cultural Norms and Definitions in the Medical Culture of Sexuality

Depictions of the insane rest on the distance between the 'sane' observer and the 'insane' subject. This is reinforced by the use of the 'beautiful' and the 'ugly' as the aesthetic norms that underscore the abyss between the observer and the subject. This intellectual rationale is rarely without specific social consequences. In an afterward to Jules Héricourt's turn-of-the-century study of 'social disease', his British translator Bernard Miall provided the reader with the ultimate rationale for the control and exclusion of the sick from the body politic. It is not only the need to separate the healthy from the sick, but equally one to isolate the beautiful from the ugly:

We need a religion of beauty, of perfection. It would be a simple matter to teach children to worship perfection rather than hate it because it reveals their own imperfection. For we cannot teach what beauty is without making plain the hideousness of egoism. Beauty is the outward and visible sign of health – perfection – virtue. Pleasure is the perception of beauty, or some of its elements. What makes for the fullness and perfection of life, for beauty and happiness, is good; what makes for death, disease, imperfection, suffering, is bad. These things are capable of proof, and a child may understand them. Sin is ugly and painful. Perfection is beautiful and gives us joy. We have appealed to the Hebraic conscience for two thousand years in vain. Let us appeal to the love of life and beauty which is innate in all of us. A beauty-loving people could not desire to multiply a diseased or degenerate strain, or hate men and women because they were strong and comely and able. . . . The balance of the races is overset, and only the abandonment of voluntary sterility by the fit, and its adoption by the unfit – which is eugenics – can save us.[1]

Miall's view echoes an association of the healthy with the beautiful that acquired its most explicit statement at the close of the nineteenth century. It is not only that the healthy becomes the beautiful, but that the beautiful becomes the healthy; the diseased is not only the ugly, but the ugly the diseased.[2] And the ugly must be made to give way to the beautiful through the agency of scientific medicine. What is desired is a world peopled by the beautiful, and only an absolute norm of beauty is permitted.

The association of the beautiful and the healthy is as ancient as Hippocrates. One must remember the age-old tradition that the physician must appear healthy. Hippocrates opens his description of *The Physician* with the observation that 'the dignity of a physician requires that he should look healthy, and as plump as nature intended him to be; for the common crowd consider those who are not of excellent bodily condition to be unable to take care of others'.[3] This tradition dominates even the modern view of the physician in which the doctor must have 'a sound constitution and a healthy look, which indeed seem as necessary qualifications for a physician as a good life and virtuous behaviour for a divine'.[4] Beauty, morals and character are all intertwined with the notion of being able to do good, but also in being good. Even Milton's description in *Paradise Lost* of the effects of the Fall on physiognomy and character is in terms of erotic health and illness:

> 'Their Maker's image', answered Michael, 'then
> Forsook them, when themselves they vilified
> To serve ungoverned appetite, and took
> His image whom they served, a brutish vice,
> Inductive mainly to the sin of Eve.
> Therefore so abject is their punishment,
> Disfiguring not God's likeness, but their own,
> Or of his likeness, by themselves defaced
> While they pervert pure Nature's healthful rules
> To loathsome sickness; worthily, since they
> God's image did not reverence in themselves.'[5]

By the eighteenth century the association of the beautiful and the good is simply accepted in the philosophical discourse of the time. For Kant, as in the *Critique of Aesthetic Judgment*, they are closely interrelated categories, as both the 'beautiful' and the 'good' please the self.[6]

But if the beautiful and the good were linked, their antithesis in the aesthetics of the age was not only the ugly and the evil. By the mid-nineteenth century Karl Rosenkranz, Hegel's best-known student, justified his undertaking an aesthetics of the ugly by stating in his introduction that the study of the ugly is to the examination of beauty as the study of pathology is to illness.[7] The medical analogy – the exploration of the dead body as a means to understand the living one, or of the ugly body to understand the beautiful one – is central to his analysis, as the pathological came to be understood as the ugly. Illness, deformity, loss of function, ageing, malproportion, infection, risk – all the categories that in medical thought defined deviancy from the healthy norm become one with the notion of the ugly. In Rosenkranz's aesthetics of the ugly, the 'ugly' is dependent on the essential nature 'beauty'. 'Beauty', like 'goodness', for him, is an absolute category; 'ugliness', like 'evil', is a relative one. Likewise, illness is understood in the medical (and pathological) literature of the nineteenth century as dependent in its definition on the definition of the normal.[8] The healthy are the baseline for any definition of the acceptable human being, as if the changes of the body, labelled as illness or ageing or disability, were foreign to the definition of the 'real' human being.

However, Rosenkranz, in deriving the ugly as ultimately from the transcendental concept of the beautiful, provided a rather striking loophole. Indeed, he noted, if the antithesis of the ugly as the 'negative-beautiful' could be eliminated, the ugly could again become part of the world of beauty. Even the ugly, therefore, can please. Here the problem of the attraction of the ugly (and, by extension, the ill) is raised in its intensity. Why is the observer fascinated as well as repelled by the image of illness?

Rosenkranz contrasts this potential liberation of the ugly with the realities of its meaning within a world of illness. Indeed, his comments on the aesthetics of illness document, as well as Kant's views, the presuppositions from which the Western aestheticization of illness departs. Ugliness is the embodiment of evil (*das Böse*) as an abstraction. Such ugliness can be seen as a response to 'the specific location in which it is found' in the body of the Black (*der Neger*) or as a specific response to illness, as in the scrofulous. Thus Rosenkranz sees the body of the Black as ugly, but not as ugly as the body of the cretin (the touchstone for discussion of degeneration at mid-century), for the latter (p. 32) adds 'stupidity of intelligence and weakness of spirit'.[9] Here racial categories come to have parallel, if not identical, meanings to labels of illness. For Rosenkranz goes on to argue that 'if the human being, like the Bushman or the cretin, is ugly by nature, this form establishes itself in their inheritance'. Thus ugliness becomes a category to delineate the healthy from the ill through its persistent potential across time and generations.

These images of inherited ugliness and illness move Rosenkranz in the very same paragraph to define what specifically makes the body ugly in the course of illness. 'Illness', according to Rosenkranz, 'is the source of ugliness when it alters the form of the body'. Not surprisingly, he stresses those illnesses that 'dye the skin' and his prime example is syphilis, as it not only marks the skin but creates the 'most ghastly deformities' (p. 33). But there is a counter-disease for Rosenkranz, one that in its 'emaciation, its pale cheeks or its cheeks reddened by fever makes the spirit immediately evident' (p. 33). This is tuberculosis. 'Who would have not seen the transfigured gaze of a young woman or young man on their deathbeds, victims of tuberculosis! This is impossible for animals.' But this is not beauty for Rosenkranz. That only comes with the restitution of health – 'the eventual return of health gives the gaze a true clarity, the cheeks a soft blush' (p. 34). This is health – tuberculosis only mimics it and thus provides a false image of the beautiful.

Here the fascination with the diseased is posed as an aesthetic problem. But it is answered by the assumption that an aesthetics of beauty can be transcultural. For Kant or Rosenkranz the norms of the beautiful/ugly – like the norms of the healthy/ill – are not bound to any culture. Therefore disease too forms a universal category of aesthetic evaluation. In his discussion Rosenkranz focuses on the deformed as his category of the diseased. The deformed is that structure of human existence which deviates from the norm of the beautiful (i.e., functional) body. Given Rosenkranz's position at the mid-point of the nineteenth century, just as B. A. Morel was formulating the notion of 'degeneration', it should be of little surprise that the aesthetics of the ugly and the diseased became a type of aesthetic degeneration theory. The existence of an a priori notion of the beautiful allows a limited number of possibilities for the existence of the ugly, just as the existence of an a priori notion of the healthy presents a limited range of possibilities for the existence of the diseased.

The dichotomy between the beautiful and the ugly seems to be inherent in all of the cultural constructs of health and disease in the nineteenth and twentieth centuries. Miall's statement is made in defining the ultimate of horrors for the turn of the century physician – the 'social diseases' – under which the author of the volume, Jules Héricourt, understands syphilis, tuberculosis, alcoholism and sterility. These 'illnesses' are not only deviations from an absolute aesthetic norm, they 'disfigure' the body politic through the 'infection' of the individual. By the end of the nineteenth century individual beauty comes to have significance as a sign of the healthiness of the race. Here, to no-one's surprise, the notion of the healthy and beautiful race has evolved into the discourse of eugenics. It is only the 'new' science, here eugenics, that can restore the beauty of the body politic. 'Race', however, is only a place-holder for the idea of the 'healthy' and 'beautiful' collective that must be preserved.

And the antithesis to this new vocabulary of aesthetic perfection is, according to Miall, the old and faulty promise of conscience and religion, with its 'Hebraic conscience'. In starkly Nietzschean terms, Miall defines the brave new world of European (defined as British if you are in Britain; German if you are in Germany; French if you are in France) science against Christianity, the legacy of the Jews in Europe. This move is not an accidental one. With the rise of materialism within medicine, the struggle comes to be between 'theology' (ugly) and 'science' (beauty), and Nietzsche reads this as an overcoming of the Jewish (read ugly) aspect of the modern soul. The Jew is the very model of the ugly and the diseased (illus. 20). Nietzsche argued in *The Genealogy of Morals* (1887) that it was 'the Jew who, with frightening consistency, dared to invert the aristocratic value equations good/ noble/powerful/beautiful/happy/favored-of-the-god and maintain that only the poor, the powerless, are good; only the suffering, sick, and ugly, truly blessed'.[10] The second half of this quotation is, of course, a summary of the Beatitudes, for Christianity is merely Rabbinic Judaism in another guise. It is the weak, sickly and ugly race that must give way to its antithesis, the strong, the healthy, the beautiful.

When translated into the discourse of the favoured versus the ill-favoured races, one major aspect of the aesthetics of health and illness surfaces. It is the association of the beautiful with the erotic; the ugly with the unerotic. The unerotic or the unpleasurable must give way to the pleasure of the erotic. It is the attraction of the beautiful that will enable the race to maintain its beauty. These terms are unmistakably gendered. Thus in Héricourt's terms sterility is a social disease that makes the female, no matter how alluring on the surface, inherently ugly. Only the fecund are truly beautiful for they reproduce the race. For in the discourse of health, the erotic comes to play a major role in defining what is beautiful and what ugly.

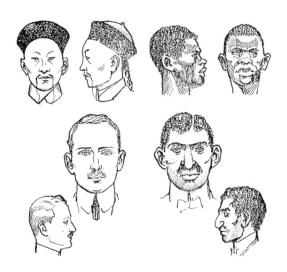

20 Jews and other 'ugly' races, in contrast to the 'normal' Aryan. From Karl Paumgartten, *Juda* (Graz, n.d.).

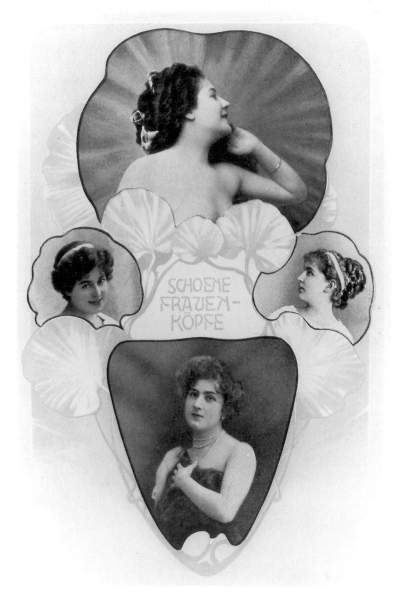

21 Anna Fischer-Duckelmann's images of the healthy and therefore beautiful female, from her *Die Frau als Hausärztin* (Stuttgart, 1911).

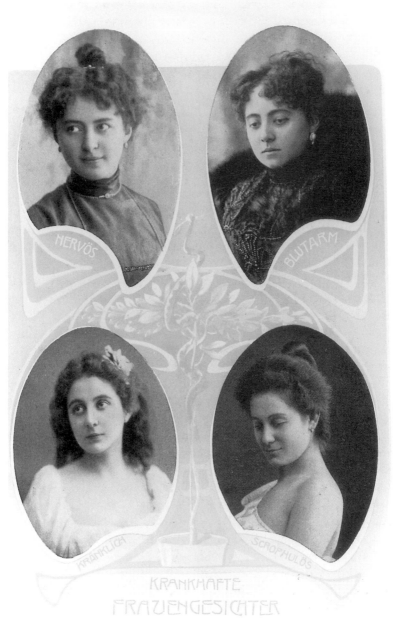

22 Fisher-Duckelmann's images of the ill and therefore ugly female; clockwise from top left: nervous, anaemic, scrofulous, fragile; from her *Die Frau als Hausärztin*.

In her handbook of health for woman at the *fin de siècle*, Anna Fischer-Duckelmann presents two images contrasting the erotically healthy and the ill body, the beautiful and the ugly body in terms of reproductive function (illus. 21, 22).[11] Fischer-Duckelmann stands in a long medical tradition of associating female health and beauty, positive reproductive capacities and the maintenance or improvement of the race.[12] What is important in her work is that like many physicians indebted to aesthetic theories of physiognomy at the turn of the century, she provides the reader/viewer with a visual vocabulary in order to establish her theoretical positions. Her views extend those of the eighteenth-century physiognomists, such as Lavater, whose initial ideas were rooted in medical physiognomy and who extended them into every possible arena of race and gender. And since the very idea of the 'beautiful' draws on the status of sight as the highest, most rational and purest sense, visual proof is the most effective manner of making her case. In her work the visual representation of the physiognomy of health/beauty (at least women's health) and the physiognomy of illness/ugliness compete for attention within identical frames. But one can read the difference in the physiognomies of those who will be reproductively more efficient and productive. Not only are the 'healthy' women plumper (like Hippocrates' doctor), but, one can note, they also have a lighter complexion and are 'happier' in terms of their expression. 'Ill' people are not only 'bad' people, they are also 'unhappy' people.

When Fischer-Duckelmann presents the ideal female body type, she invokes a 'classical' image of beauty taken from late nineteenth-century German internalizations of Greek beauty. And it is clearly associated with the state of the psyche. For nineteenth-century Germans, after the reception of the classics through the work of Winckelmann, Greek beauty becomes German beauty. This Græco-German beauty is defined as a serenity of the spirit. The 'beautiful' construction of the body and the visage came to be a constant in late nineteenth-century medicine. The noted Viennese physiologist Ernst Brücke, one of Freud's teachers, published a handbook of the anatomical 'beauty' of the body in 1891. Brücke, who had been a lecturer in anatomy at the Berlin Academy of Arts, presented a normative body based on classical aesthetics. Thus he invokes Michelangelo's representation of the female breast in positing the perfect breast (illus. 23), or the classical line of Diadumenos for the perfect male torso (illus. 24). The perfect female body seems to be the pubescent body, unmarked by childbirth, but prepared for it; the perfect male body is also unmarked, not least by circumcision. What is clear in Brücke's image of the beautiful is that it draws on ideal notions of 'classical' perfection, but uses it to stress the

23 The perfect female breast, from Ernst Brücke, *Schönheit und Fehler der menschlichen Gestalt* (Vienna, 1891).

24 The perfect male torso (penis uncircumcised of course), from Brücke's *Schönheit und Fehler der menschlichen Gestalt*.

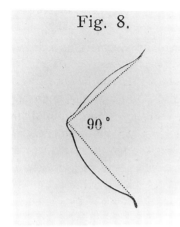

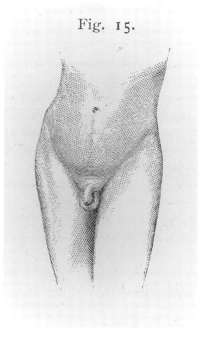

values of contemporary society. The aesthetics of high art were, according to Brücke's assumption, rooted in an idea of art as mimesis. Works of art imitated the most beautiful human beings, rather than created ideal types. Thus even in foot and leg positions, Brücke presents what is the 'real' image of the beautiful: the beautiful foot is not the flat foot, at least according to him.[13] The flat foot, as I have shown in detail elsewhere, is the foot of the Black and the Jew in *fin de siècle* European medicine, a foot that disqualifies the possessor from ever being fully a citizen of the modern European state.[14] The idealized image of the beautiful is also the image of the healthy.

And these qualities are often located explicitly in the definition of feminine beauty. Thus the question of character ('serenity'), body form ('plumpness'), and skin colour ('lightness') become signs of reproductive and racial health. Kant recognizes these categories as early as his essay on the Sublime, when he writes concerning the nature of female beauty that the beautiful woman is defined by 'a well proportioned figure, regular features, colours of eyes and face which contrast prettily, beauties pure and simple which are also pleasing in a bouquet and gain a cool approbation'. This 'beauty' is reflected in the character of the woman, for 'the moral composition makes itself discernible in the mien or facial features, she whose features show qualities of beauty is *agreeable*, and if she is that to a high degree, *charming*.[15] Implied in Kant's argument is 'youthfulness', which defines the erotic. If, as he argues, the female defines the beautiful, the link between beauty and health (defined as reproductive ability) is clear. Only the beautiful should be able to, or would want to, reproduce.

Such beauty is universal: 'I affirm that the sort of beauty we have called the pretty figure is judged by all men very much alike. . . . The Turks, the Arabs, the Persians are apparently of one mind in this taste, because they are very eager to beautify their races through such fine blood [of Circassian and Georgian maidens]' (p. 89). The cultural significance of these views in late nineteenth-century Europe is clear.[16] It is not only that these physical signs of difference are taken to have diagnostic value. That which is 'ill-proportioned, irregular, non-contrastive' is not only ill, but will make a society as a whole ill. From the eighteenth century, those defined as 'not German' in Germany, such as the Jews, are seen as having darker or yellowish skin colour and, as we shall see, often are labelled as having a body form that reveals their potential for illness.

By the nineteenth century, male Jews are seen as feminized, belonging to an 'inferior race'.[17] The Jew, in his 'absence of creative power, of spontaneity and of originality . . . displays in this respect something of a woman's nature. The Semites are said to be a feminine race, possessing to a high degree the gift of receptivity, always lacking in virility and procreative power' (p. 247). The visualization of the difference of the male Jew is thus in terms of this image of the unproductive and the ill, specifically the image of the tubercular female, who is simultaneously 'beautiful' (but dangerous) and 'diseased'. Here Rosenkranz's image comes full circle in categorizing the apparent rejection of the Jew as a figure of desire in post-Enlightenment Europe. The Jew's 'bodily infirmity' is marked by the Jew's 'unmanly appearance'. He is like, but not identical to, the tubercular woman, specifically the tubercular Jewish woman. The Jew's visage is like 'to those lean actresses, the *Rachels* and *Sarahs*, who spit blood, and seem to have but the spark of life left, and yet who, when they have stepped upon the stage, put forth indomitable strength and energy. Life, with them, has hidden springs' (p. 150). It is the tubercular Jewish woman that the healthy male Jew looks like. It is Sarah Bernhardt (1844–1923) and Rachel Félix (1820–58), the two best-known Jewish actresses on the nineteenth-century Paris stage, both tubercular, who mark the essence of the normal physiognomy of the *male* Jew. Jewish women, for example, are rarely considered to be 'agreeable' or 'charming'.

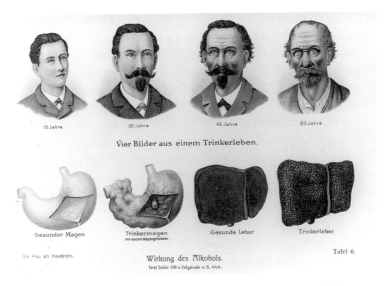

15 Jahre 30 Jahre 45 Jahre 60 Jahre

Vier Bilder aus einem Trinkerleben.

Gesunder Magen Trinkermagen Gesunde Leber Trinkerleber
mit rundem Magengeschwür.

Die Frau als Hausärztin.

Wirkung des Alkohols.
Text Seite 110 u.folgende u.S. 440.

Tafel 6.

25 The decay of the beautiful body through alcohol; and a comparison of the 'healthy' and 'drinker's' liver and stomach. From Fischer-Duckelmann's *Die Frau als Hausärztin*.

And yet why is it, Kant asks, that 'many women' have a liking for 'a healthy but pale colour', which should, he implies, be a sign of pathology? 'This generally accompanies a disposition of more inward feeling and delicate sensation, which belongs to the quality of the Sublime; where as the rosy and blooming complexion proclaims less of the first, but more of the joyful and merry disposition – but it is more suitable to vanity to move and to arrest, than to charm and to attract' (p. 88). Again it is character that is mirrored in the face. But it is not the face of the pathological, only that which evokes or affirms the possibility of that which is greater than the self, the Sublime. The aesthetic qualities often ascribed to the ill ('delicacy') come to signal a type of character that is merely a variation on the beautiful, rather than its antithesis. But this problem of distinguishing between the truly sick and the truly healthy, the truly beautiful and the truly ugly, is never resolved by the philosophers of the age.

The simple dichotomy of the 'beautiful' as opposed to the 'ugly' is gendered in Fischer-Duckelmann's association of the antithesis of female beauty. In her image of the physiognomy of the (male) alcoholic a similar contrast – here over time – can be observed (illus. 25). Here the 'healthy' and 'beautiful' male, destined to become an alcoholic, reveals his nature in his physiognomy as certainly as in his organs. Here the mask of the normal is revealed to be a mask by the effects of a degenerate life over time. This displacement is interesting as it

61

presents a case of gender reversal. In male medical writers the trope of decay is most often associated with the female; in this text written by a woman for women, the image of the decaying alcoholic is a male. Beauty, therefore, can be true beauty when associated by Fischer-Duckelmann with the female and her reproductive capacities, but when associated with the image of the male it reveals itself to be false beauty. For the alcoholic will damage not only his own being but will translate his degeneracy into damage for the race.

In the general medical literature on degeneracy, the signs of beauty and ugliness are usually gendered in quite a different manner. 'Plumpness', as I have shown elsewhere, had a double-edged meaning at the turn of the century: it was a sign of stability but also, potentially, a sign of satiety and sexuality. 'Normal' women, to use Cesare Lombroso's distinction, can be plump and are therefore healthy; 'criminal women, such as prostitutes' are plump, a sign of their 'natural' tendency to their craft. It is important to note that the contexts for the reading of the physiognomy are absolutely clear – one knows whether the sign of plumpness means danger or succour. But chronologically, and here the notion of degeneracy again rears its head, it is impossible to tell. We know, says Lombroso's Russian colleague Pauline Tarnowsky, that even the most beautiful prostitute will eventually reveal her degenerate physiognomy, for what is within must out.[18]

Certainly this image of beauty as the mask of a dangerous – i.e., infectious or contagious – illness has affected the representation of the body of the tubercular in the nineteenth and twentieth centuries. So there has been a need to unmask the hidden pathology under the skin. Thus questions of 'constitution' and 'body type' attempt to reveal the hidden illness well before the illness manifests itself. No clearer pattern for the relationship between an idealized body type and an 'ugly', i.e. potentially ill, body type can be found than in the ancient question of whether people with a specific body type are predisposed to acquiring tuberculosis. The *habitus phthisicus* was the clearest sign for an 'inherited diathesis', a predisposition to tuberculosis, as early as the times of Hippocrates and Galen. Indeed, in the eighteenth century Friedrich Hoffmann believed that 'tall people with long necks' were prone to tuberculosis.[19] This tradition of the ugly as a sign of disease is stressed in the classic history of constitutional theory that opened the standard *fin de siècle* periodical on the topic.[20] The ugly may not be immediately ill, but their deformed bodies predispose them to illness (illus. 26, 27). They hide within them the roots of the destruction of the collective, because if they reproduce their body type will predispose their offspring to illness.

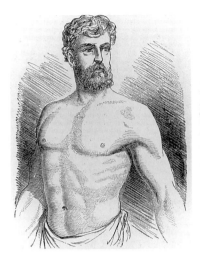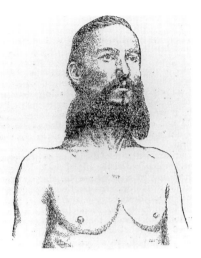

26 The healthy chest of a 'real' man.   27 The *habitus phthisicus* of a 'weakling'.
From Paul Niemeyer, *The Lungs in Health and Disease* (London, 1908).

The classic nineteenth-century description of this 'ugly body', the *habitus phthisicus*, was that of Christoph Wilhelm Hufeland (1762–1836), which stressed that 'the constitutional consumption [the *habitus phthisicus*, called by Hufeland the *phthisis constitutionalis*], innate in the organism by structure, heredity, and the corporeal disposition, endeavours through the whole period of life to develop itself; it can be delayed, but never entirely annihilated, and once developed, is incurable.' The physical form of the *phthisis constitutionalis* was linked by Hufeland with the character of the predisposed individual. The *phthisis constitutionalis* was understood

to be marked by a flat thorax, narrow towards the side and back, shoulder blades protruding wing-like, long neck, slender body, and very white teeth, but above all, by a peculiar irritability of the vascular system and lungs; thence circumscribed red cheeks (called phthisical roses), appearing especially after eating, easily excited, over-heating and redness of the face on rising, hot hands after meals, cough easily excited; irritable, sanguine temper, but particularly by an indifference and a carelessness of their own health, especially concerning that of the lungs, so that they entirely overlook, in reporting their case, the difficulties in the lungs, or pass them over intentionally, and attribute their disease generally to some other part, especially to the abdomen.[21]

Here the notion of character (sanguinity) and body type as a sign of potential illness are linked. The ill individual is by definition someone whose character or psyche is also ill. This asymmetry, ill-proportion, irregularity can be easily contrasted to Kant's idealized body, with its pseudo-Greek colour, balance and proportion.

63

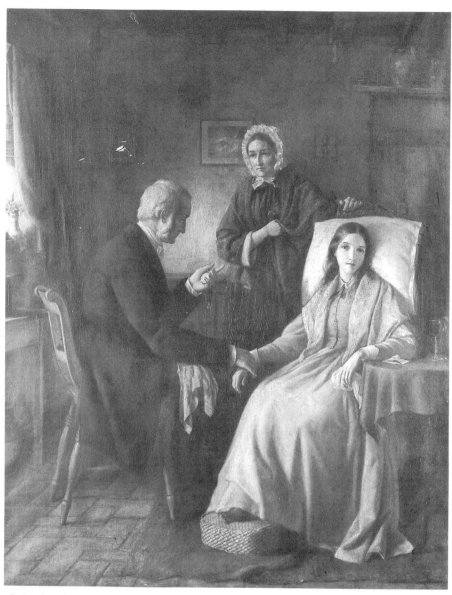

28 Attributed to E. Kennedy, *Fading Away*, oil on canvas, loosely based on Henry
Peach Robinson's famous photograph of 1857 with the same title. London, The
Wellcome Institute for the History of Medicine.

The turn of the century image of the *habitus phthisicus* presented an 'ugly' body type, always associated with racial types such as the Jews. Marriage of an Aryan with a Jew would introduce a 'diseased' character marked by a recognizable, deformed body into a pure race and cause the latter to degenerate. It is within the model of degeneration that Albert Reibmayr places the problem of the marriage of the tubercular.[22] For Reibmayr it is the *habitus phthisicus*, the physical body of the person with tuberculosis, that signals the decline of the 'original racial type'. Here the bad body, the *habitus phthisicus*, drives out the good racial body, as the race becomes more and more predisposed to tuberculosis. The changes in the body caused by the tubercular bacilli are inherited by successive generations.

Tuberculosis marked the body as different, even in the seemingly attractive fantasy of the female tubercular (illus 28), as in the *Lady of the Camellias* by Dumas *fils*, set to music in Verdi's *Traviata*, or Murger's Mimi, set to music in Puccini's *Bohème*. There, too, sexual contact with one may have been allowed across the abyss of class or race, but reproduction, as Miall warns, had to be prevented. Rosenkranz's view that such 'beauty' was merely false beauty reappears within these stories. In each there is a moment of seeming recuperation in which the 'healthiness' of the individuals with tuberculosis merely masks the continuing presence of the illness. Reproduction is therefore impossible if Rosenkranz's mid-century reading is valid: such illnesses and their aesthetic markers will be passed from generation to generation. A tubercular patient's desire to have children would be understood at the time as a sign of psychopathology: 'The tubercular patient often loses an understanding that he out of various reasons cannot partake of the joys of love and should not place any more children into the world. He stomps on these general hygienic as well as eugenic, aesthetic and sociological premises . . .'.[23] Here, in the words of a medical specialist of the day, concepts are linked that have been assumed but hitherto not articulated. For it is not only eugenic (purity of the race), hygienic (purity of the individual) and sociological (purity of the society) concerns that should make a tubercular individual hesitant to have offspring, but also aesthetic ones. Here the world of the 'beautiful' – of the creation of the work of art – is evoked. The tubercular body is unaesthetic and will produce ugly (i.e., diseased) children, and thus the race will be at risk. The earlier evocation of the tubercular Jewish woman as the marker of the sick Jew associated the danger to the race with the danger of disease. Race mixing is thus seen as dangerous as infection. This trope is yet a newer version of an ancient set of associations reaching back into the Middle Ages.[24]

The dichotomy is clear: The healthy is the beautiful, is the erotic, is the good, for it leads to the preservation and continuation of the collective. This is the norm against which the deviant is to be measured. The deviant is ill and is therefore ugly and evil. (Being ill, the degenerate is excluded because of the danger to the collective.) The ugliness of the deviant may be overtly evident upon first glance, may appear over time, or may be evident only to the 'trained eye' of the physician/aesthetician. That which is ill is therefore inherently anti-erotic, even though it may mask itself as the 'false' or pseudo-erotic. The true erotic is connected to the world of the healthy and the reproductive. The false erotic is destructive rather than reproductive as it provides no continuation of the group. There is no bridge in this model between the healthy and the ill, for illness is the antithesis or absence of health. There are no intermediate or transitional stages, only masks that are lifted to reveal the antithesis of the healthy. This resembles the model of the parasite that is applied to pariah groups, including the ill, during this period. The ill are predisposed to their state or they embody it, or they only mask healthiness and the erotic. They belong to a separate world, a dangerous world that is always attempting to colonize the world of the healthy.

The notion that the beautiful body is the healthy body is the theme of the creation of the New Man during the late nineteenth and early twentieth centuries. This New Man (and New Woman) is seen as the natural improvement of the species through the alteration of the social system. These new systems produce not only better citizens, it was believed, but more beautiful ones. This view can be found in various national movements of the early twentieth century, from Italian fascism to Zionism. George Mosse has established the subtle national differences among these 'new' men and women.[25] These idealized body types are paralleled by ideal 'moral' types, by 'good citizens'. The beautiful citizen is the good citizen; the healthy citizen is the good citizen. And citizenship in this context is a reflex of the body. The good citizen cannot be ugly and therefore cannot be infected by, or infect, members of society with dangerous illnesses, illnesses that would be marked on their physiognomies.

4 The Phantom of the Opéra's Nose

The syphilitic is not the good citizen. In the age of infection syphilis is ugly, but the syphilitic him- or herself may hide behind a mask of beauty, much like the tubercular woman. This will, however, eventually reveal itself to be but a mask. Even the public health posters announcing the syphilitic as the potential source of infection to the body politic (illus. 29) may themselves represent the syphilitic as beautiful, and the erotic is but a trap to deceive and destroy. Nowhere is this link between the disease and the erotic more evidently worked out than in Gaston Leroux's novel of 1911, *The Phantom of the Opéra*. Here the 'mask' is truly only a mask and the image of the diseased gives the reader access to the problem of the erotic and the visibility of the ugly.

'The Opéra ghost really existed', or so Leroux claimed at the very beginning of his novel. In a true sense the Opéra ghost really did exist – at least the horror that the hidden face of the Phantom evoked was quite real to Leroux's readers both then and since.

What was it about the potential sight of Erik, the Phantom of the Opéra, that so terrified (and fascinated) Leroux's audience? As readers we are given glimpses of the Phantom's face through the eyes of members of the Opéra very early in the book, and these are frightening. His masked face had

eyes . . . so deep that you can hardly see the fixed pupils. You just see two big black holes, as in a dead man's skull. His skin, which is stretched across his bones like a drumhead, is not white, but a nasty yellow. His nose is so little worth talking about that you can't see it side-face; and the absence of that nose is a horrible thing to look at.[1]

This missing nose seems to be the locus of the horror felt by the viewers, but also by the Phantom himself. He often sports a 'long, thin, and transparent' nose that is evidently 'a false nose' (p. 30). 'When he went out in the streets or ventured to show in public, he wore a pasteboard nose, with a moustache attached to it, instead of his own horrible hole of a nose. This did not quite take away his corpse-like air, but it made him almost, I say almost, endurable to look at' (p. 207). His

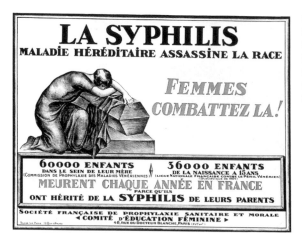

29 Hereditary syphilis assassinates the race, according to a French poster of the 1920s on the degeneration of the race.

missing nose leads him to hate those with 'real noses' (p. 227). And this missing nose gave his face the aura of a death's head. Indeed, the ghost 'smelt of death' (p. 126). He felt himself as 'built up of death from head to foot' with 'his terrible dead flesh' (p. 129).

The essence of the Phantom – his unrequited love for the soprano Christine Daaé, the singer he tutors and eventually abandons – is built around the horrid aspect of his face. What does the mask conceal? We see his face very early on in the novel, and its very physiognomy reveals that which is at the centre of Erik's horror: branded on his physiognomy are the scars of congenital syphilis. The missing nose, the fixed pupils, the stench of rotting flesh are all (at least in the popular mind of the turn of the century) indicators of the social disease that marks him. And the medical physiognomists of the turn of the century, such as Byrom Bramwell, froze these faces in their textbooks for all to examine (illus. 30). The Phantom's own horror at his obsessive love for Christine Daaé, his desire for consummation of his love and his rejection of it, is rooted in the repugnance he feels toward his own body. His artificial nose is a sign that contemporary readers would have understood to be a visible mark of his disease. But Erik's illness was not of his making: he was born malformed, 'his ugliness a subject of horror and terror to his parents' (p. 261). Their horror pointed to the social stigmatization of their own sexuality, visible now for everyone to see in the deformity of their son.

The erotic and reproduction are linked for the turn of the century in the concept of hereditary syphilis. The missing nose represents a castration, not merely as an attenuated *fin de siècle* metaphor, but as a real action: not only social castration, but the inherent undesirability that infected people should reproduce. Eric is the product of individ-

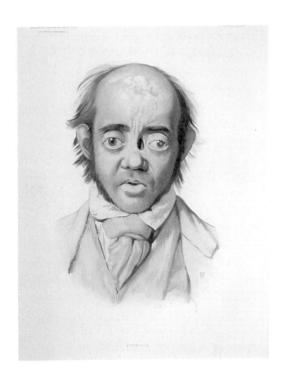

30 The marked face of the syphilitic, from Byrom Bramwell's *Atlas of Clinical Medicine* (Edinburgh, 1894).

uals whose sexuality was polluted and whose pollution is proven by the deformity of their child. It is the phallus that is represented here as infected, not the vagina. But the opposite is the case in the sickly child of the prostitute Nana, whose death is recorded in Zola's eponymous novel. Such individuals cannot be erotically attractive, since to be attractive would be a sign of the potential, even the desirability, for reproduction. The hidden sexual pollution of the parents inscribes itself as deformity on the body of the children.

And yet the fright generated by the masked Phantom of the Opéra, from the dread which captured moviegoers seeing the 1925 silent film starring Lon Chaney to theatregoers attending Andrew Lloyd Webber's musical of the 1980s, is the horror of that which lay under the mask: What does Erik look like? What is striking is that the question which should immediately occur to the viewer – whether now or at the turn of the century – is why Erik did not have his face rebuilt. Why is it, that at the very moment when reconstructive surgery had become aesthetic surgery, at the moment when the reconstituting of the body became an adjunct to the healing of the mind, does a novel about deformity come to capture the attention of all of Europe? Leroux wrote his novel exactly at that moment in history when the possibility of aesthetic surgery was becoming widely acknowledged. But he writes the novel as an historical one – looking back at the 1880s and the reign of the Opéra ghost; looking back at an age in which such surgery was still fraught with both danger and pain. *The Phantom of the Opéra* is thus a novel in which the promises of 'modern' life have not yet been fulfilled.

The technology of destruction was in place. Erik could threaten to demolish the Paris Opéra with his kegs of black powder. But the technology of reconstruction was not yet popularly accepted. The tensions about the promise of a new life in a new age and the destructive forces of the old century play themselves out in the physiognomy of the Opéra's Phantom and his potential for redemption. It is not divine redemption that is the focus of this work, but the impossibility of any human intervention that could truly redeem the protagonist. In the 1880s no medicine could cure Erik, and his very visage evoked a specific world of horror and disease. Erik is not John Merrick ('The Elephant Man'), whose deformities could be the subject both of Victorian curiosity and charity. Merrick's deformed face evoked pity; Erik's face, the face of the syphilitic, evoked the horror of contagion.[2] Merrick became deformed; Erik's deformity was evident at birth. It is no wonder that the very aetiology of the Phantom of the Opéra's deformity shifts over time. Rupert Julien's American film, with Chaney as the Phantom, repeats Leroux's aetiology (illus. 31): Chaney adapts the standard physiognomy of hereditary syphilis for his make-up. His careful make-up representing Erik's missing nose was a sign of the diseased soul. By the time of Arthur Lubin's film (1943), with Claude Rains as Erik, the rationale for Erik's disfigurement is quite different. He has been scarred by acid thrown at him by the man he employed to engrave the score of his opera. His face *becomes* scarred; he was not born disfigured.

Not surprisingly, it was medicine that was associated with the 'healing' of such damaged visages. Even Nikolai Gogol, in his black fantasy of 1836, could have his Major Kovalyov, who awoke one morning without his nose, be given the reminder to 'see a doctor about it. I've heard there's a certain kind of specialist who can fix you up with any kind of nose you like'.[3] Edgar Allan Poe could ironically propose his own reading of the nose in 'Lionizing', his 1835 satire of social climbing, in which the 'greatness of the [social] lion is in proportion to the size of his proboscis', and in which the greatest social error is to lose one's nose.[4] For the missing nose was a most visible sign of social failure. Poe's pun is clear – he calls the 'science of the nose' in his kingdom of Bluddennuff, his satirized German pocket principality à la Voltaire, 'nosology', the technical term for the structure of the study of

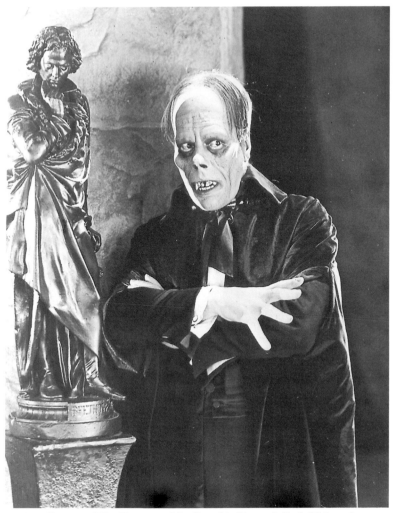

31 Lon Chaney as 'The Phantom of the Opera' in Rupert Julien's Universal Studios film of 1925.

diseases (p. 212). And indeed, Walter de la Mare's 1925 ironic fantasy of Sam Such, the little boy who came to believe that his nose was wax, presents quite the opposite of Gogol's dilemma: his parent's belief in the child's supposed infirmity made the child into a recluse and social misfit; one could not go out in public with a wax nose.[5] But it was a physician who inadvertently 'cured' his patient by placing him before a roaring fire, which did not melt his 'wax' nose. In both case the image of the 'false nose' evoked a deep-seated anxiety about disease and its implication. And in all cases it is the psychological state of the characters that is the centre of the attention.

The concern about the continuation and integrity of the 'group' is also written on the nose. In William Saroyan's *The Human Comedy* (1943), the central chapter in the education of the protagonist is called 'A Speech on the Human Nose'. In it, Homer Macauley holds a speech on the centrality of the nose to human history: 'The nose is perhaps the most ridiculous part of the human face. It has always been a source of embarrassment to the human race, and the Hittites probably beat up on everybody because their noses were so big and crooked.'[6] Thus the notion of the 'unhappy' psyche marked by the ugly nose that evokes disease is moved into the world of race and politics. Saroyan's intent is not to prove that difference is written on the face by the nose but rather to stress the universality of all human experience: 'People all over the world have noses' (p. 62). And thus the racial implications of the nose are undercut in the chapter in the following exchange:

'Moses was in the Bible,' Henry said.
'Did he have a nose?' Joe said.
'Sure he had a nose,' Henry said.
'All right, then,' Joe said. 'Why don't you say, "Moses had a nose as big as most noses?' This is an ancient history class. Why don't you try to learn something once in a while? Moses-noses-ancient-history. Catch on?'
Henry tried to catch on. 'Moses noses,' he said. 'No, wait a minute. Moses's nose was a big nose.'
'Ah,' Joe said, 'You'll never learn anything. You'll die in the poorhouse. Moses had a nose as big as most noses!' (pp. 65–6).

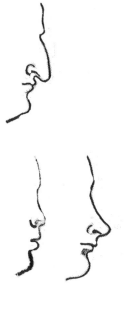

32 George Jabet (writing as Eden Warwick), in his *Notes on Noses* (London, 1848), characterized the 'Jewish, or Hawknose' (the uppermost image, as opposed to the snub and turned-up noses) as 'very convex, and preserves its convexity like a bow, throughout the whole length from the eyes to the tip. It is thin and sharp'. Shape also carried here a specific meaning: '[it] indicates considerable Shrewdness in worldly matters; a deep insight into character, and facility of turning that insight to profitable account'.

Written at the height of Nazi attacks on the Jews, Saroyan's novel is a novel about war, death and toleration as seen from small-town California. The various systems of physiognomy that dominated popular consciousness during the late nineteenth and early twentieth centuries associated bad character with big noses and saw both in the image of the Jew (illus. 32). Saroyan's exchange evokes all the claims for a difference written on the face, a difference that marks the superior from the inferior, and ironically destroys them. This is similar to Edmond Rostand's gesture in his *Cyrano de Bergerac*, in which good character and a large nose are associated. Written in 1897, Rostand's play rejects the intense anti-Semitism of the Dreyfus affair in the portrait of the large-nosed protagonist, although Cyrano's matrimonial ambitions are nevertheless thwarted. Thus the play avoids even a hint of 'miscegenation'. 'Big noses', even those that mark a noble character, do not marry and procreate with 'normal noses', such as Roxanne.

The image of the mutilated nose disfiguring the face can serve as a further example of the central problem of this book: How the culture of medicine defines and uses the distinction between 'healthy/beauty' and 'illness/ugliness'. Why is it that only at the close of the nineteenth century does aesthetic surgery grow out of reconstructive surgery? Why do Erik or Kovalyov or Sam Such despair about their respective noses? And what would it take to make them happy? How does racial physiognomy dovetail with medical ideas of 'health/beauty' and 'illness/ugliness'? The (real or fantasized) missing or grotesque noses would have been the subject of reconstructive surgery in the course of the nineteenth century, for the missing nose would have been a pathological sign rather than an aesthetic error. Their wax noses could have been replaced by reconstructed noses. And yet what is wrong with each of them is not only inscribed on the face but also on the soul. Erik's devilish torture chamber, his murders in the Opéra, his mad fascination with his own opera based on the lover Don Juan, his unfulfilled – and perhaps unfulfillable – desire for Christine Daaé, all point to an individual whose damaged face mirrors his damaged psyche. Kovalyov's sense of 'looking like a freak' (p. 63) and Sam Such's 'dreadful secret' (p. 181) and 'solitary life' (p. 186), while not as melodramatic as the fate of the Opéra's Phantom, show the impact of their real or imagined loss on their psychic life. How you look is who you are! And if you evoke the spectre of disease and difference you are less than you can be.

What is being reconstructed by the cosmetic surgeon (or his surrogate in these texts, the novelist) is the erotic and the sensual as opposed to the visible, the ugly, the corrupt. It is the promise to reconstruct the body in order to blot out the image of disease, to restore the body, not simply functionally, but also aesthetically. And the measure of this attractiveness lies in the sense that the individual 'likes' his or her own body. You hate what society hates. If your body is marked as diseased and foul, you internalize it as unhealthy and you become 'unhappy' with it. Thus the mark of the healthy body is the happy soul – *mens sana in corpore sano* – or perhaps, closer to the reality, the mark of the unhealthy body is the sick soul – *mens non sana in corpore insano*.

To trace this trope let us begin with the work of that individual who has been made into the 'father' of plastic and aesthetic surgery – the sixteenth-century Bolognese physician Gaspare Tagliacozzi, whose classic work on plastic surgery appeared in 1597.[7] (There is, of course, a huge literature on his antecedents, his relationship to classical Indian cosmetic surgery and the use of flap grafts, but since the myth is that it is with Tagliacozzi that the story begins, let us also begin with him.[8]) Tagliacozzi's most important innovation was the development of a means of replacing the missing nose. Now, you will say, that seems a noble and evidently needed task – a person without a nose is bound to be 'unhappy' and this unhappiness could well make him or her ill (illus. 33–35).

Here the problem of reconstructive surgery versus aesthetic surgery appears at the very 'origin' of cosmetic surgery. It is clear that anyone without a nose will be unhappy, and the reconstruction of the nose will make him or her happier and therefore healthier. Tagliacozzi recognizes this. In chapter eleven of his book he discusses the means of replacing the missing nose by the use of a flap graft. But he emphasizes that this job is the job of the surgeon and its primary purpose is not cosmetic. Rather it is to restore what nature had given and chance took away. For Tagliacozzi reconstructive surgery is the restitution of the original or idealized form of the body. But even more, it 'heals the spirit and aids the mind of the patient'. How this is accomplished is never discussed. It is simply assumed that not having a nose will make one 'unhappy' and restoring it will 'heal the spirit'.

This was equally true a century later when John Bulwer, in his 1653 treatise called *Anthropometamorphosis: Man Transform'd*, catalogued a wide range of cosmetic alterations of the body from a wide range of cultures. He understood only those changes that repair the 'unnaturall and monstrous Incroachments upon the Humane forme' and return the body to its 'Naturall State'. This natural state is 'unblemished' and close to the ideal of beauty in its 'original perfection'.[9] For the physician Bulwer it is only the doctor who can undertake such

33 The missing nose.

34 The operation.

35 The nose restored.

From Gaspare Tagliacozzi,
De curtorum chirurgia
(Venice, 1597).

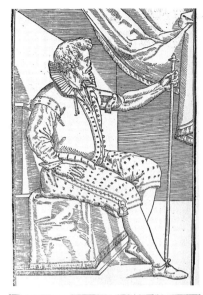

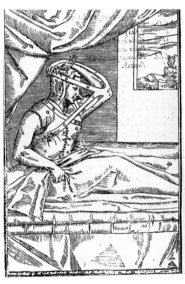

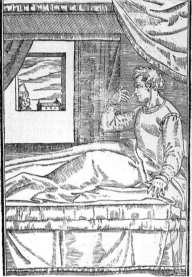

procedures on the diseased body. It is not the business of the patient or
client or even the cosmetician to repair the body. It is solely the role of
the physician or the surgeon. But, of course, in the seventeenth century
barber-surgeons not only groomed their clients but also undertook the
'removal and mitigation of marks and blemishes'.[10] In this context the
restoration of the erotic becomes the elimination of illness and disease.

Yet hidden within the views of Tagliacozzi and Bulwer is the
question of what the missing nose means, what its absence implies

about the individual. Given that evident fact that a missing nose (at least in Western culture) is a deformation, is there any further meaning which attaches itself to the nose? How does reconstituting the body with an intact nose restore the psyche? What makes the individual truly happy? Is it the invisibility of the body, looking like everyone else's, or the masking of the body's difference from everyone else's? Should the body be repaired and therefore reconstituted, even if the repair itself is noticeable and continues to mark the individual as different, or should one mask the deformity and create at least the illusion of social acceptability? What makes the person without a nose least unhappy?

One must understand that by the end of the sixteenth century the missing nose was no longer the result (if it had ever been) only of violence, on or off the battlefield or duelling ground. Rather, the missing nose became a sign of uncleanness and immorality – of the syphilitic infection that had entered Europe during the siege of Naples only a hundred years before Tagliacozzi wrote. When we turn to the world of medicine in the seventeenth century, its anxiety about sexuality, the erotic and visibility is clear, although the diagnostic categories for sexually transmitted diseases are rather less defined than later, so that scrofula and syphilis are not always understood as completely separate illnesses. But all illnesses written on the skin, following the medieval understanding of leprosy as a sexually transmitted disease, are always understood as deforming but also as making one's stigma visible.

Let us use as our example a discussion of noses in the issue of Addison and Steele's *Tatler* published on 7 December 1710.[11] Here Addison evoked a myth about Tagliacozzi's by then lost work through a quotation from Samuel Butler's *Hudibras*. Tagliacozzi, according to this legend, used not the patient's own skin, but the skin off 'the brawny Part of [the] Porter's bum', off the buttocks of the working poor, for his grafts. When they died, 'off drop'd the Sympathetick Snout'. A tale is then spun about the origin of syphilis, which led to these gentlemen needing their new noses – Cupid is born after the siege of Naples under the malevolent signs that (according to contemporary explanations) heralded the coming of the new epidemic. (Imported from the Americas, it was the Native Americans' return gift for Columbus's present of smallpox.) This Cupid 'with a sickly look and crazy constitution' shot his poisoned arrows into the lovers' noses rather than into their hearts as was his brothers' wont: he 'dipped all his Arrows in Poison, that rotten every Thing they touched; and what was more particular, aimed all of his Shafts at the Nose . . .'. These gentlemen went to the porter for their substitute noses because of the activities of

Cupid. This Cupid was sent to the 'School of Mercury, who did all he could to hinder him from demolishing the Noses of Mankind'. But this did not work and he continued to 'wound his Votaries oftner in the Nose than in the Heart'. Syphilis is not controlled, in this tale, by mercury therapy, that is by existing medicine, rather Tagliacozzi evolved a means by which he 'grafted a new [nose] on the remaining Part of the Grisle'. The doctor, according to this account, was soon overrun by those seeking to remedy the affliction visited on them by Cupid. Note that this comic tale – which has reappeared in a very different, 'post-modern', version in a rewriting by the American surgeon Richard Selzer[12] – ends with an 'Admonition to the young Men of this Town'. For today, Addison writes, there is no Tagliacozzi 'to be met with at the Corner of every Street'. The tale goes on to warn young male readers that Tagliacozzi's art has now been lost and that they should beware: 'the general Precept therefore I shall leave with them is, to regard every Town-Woman as a particular Kind of Siren, that has a Design upon their Noses, and that, amidst her Flatteries and Allurements, they will fancy she speaks to 'em in that humorous Phrase of old Plautus: "Keep your Face out of my Way, or I'll bite off your Nose".' It is from this 'distemper' which 'mutilated and disfigured his species' that Addison and Steele see Tagliacozzi's art emerging, for 'the nose is a very becoming part of the face, and a man makes but a very silly figure without it'. Such a man (and it is the man seduced by the sirens of the town that is their ideal reader) would be publicly marked by the loss of the nose. Here the erotic activities of the 'beautiful' but unclean 'Town-Woman' can lead to the destruction of male beauty. The result is a face and a body marked by syphilis.

Let us move a hundred years into the future, to the 1820s, and the discussion by a Dr von Klein about the rebuilding of the nose.[13] Procedures analogous to Tagliacozzi's had been rediscovered and reintroduced in the course of the early nineteenth century by Carl Ferdinand Graefe and J. C. Carpue. These had been 'rediscovered' in 1794 through the British colonization of India, where the flap-technique was still practiced by one of the castes as a common form of the repair of the nose. Carpue, of the York Hospital in Chelsea, described the flap procedure in 1816 as a means of repairing the syphilitic nose (illus. 36). The repair leaves, as does the Indian procedure for 'affixing a new nose on a man's face', a noticeable scar on the face, both on the roughly formed new nose and the forehead. The restoration of the nose left telltale signs of the surgery.

Dr von Klein does not advocate these procedures. They provide for him only an approximation of a real nose that 'can be seen at first

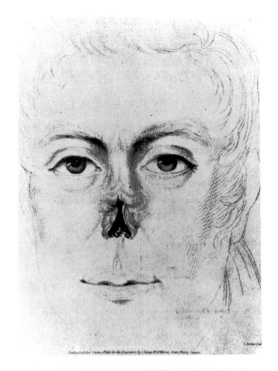

36 A soldier, suffering from a 'venereal complaint', whose nose was replaced by the flap method. From J. C. Carpue, *An Account of Two Successful Operations for Restoring a Lost Nose* (London, 1816).

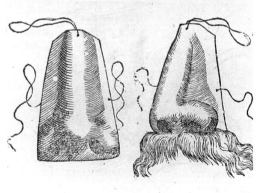

37 Ambroise Paré's artificial nose from the Renaissance. From his *Œuvres* (Paris, 1628).

glance' to be reconstructed. Rather he advocates, as did the Renaissance French surgeon, Ambroise Paré, the use of an artificial nose held on with real or imitation spectacles or a clasp (illus. 37). These imitation noses provide a more 'beautiful' nose since they are indistinguishable from the original – at least according to Dr von Klein. These noses should be made out of solid, well-carved wood and painted to match the face. Some individuals, he notes, will need a morning nose and an evening nose – the latter rather more red to match the effects of wine.

But Klein also tells us the rare story of one of his patients who requested his help in acquiring a 'more beautiful' nose. She was a young princess of less than twenty who had what is technically called a 'saddle-nose', a nose that sagged at the bridge.[14] She suggested to her physician that a bridge of gold be inserted to shape the nose so that it was straight. She suggested that this procedure first be tried on some poor individual to see whether infection and 'ugly' scarring would result. Klein proceeded to the pauper's hospital and found a male to volunteer – based on the payment of a *thaler* and the promise that he could keep the gold bridge once it was removed. To the doctor's surprise the operation was a success: no infection and a very small scar. But his original patient, the princess, vacillated once confronted with the possibility of a procedure that involved neither general nor local anaesthetics. At one point she actually got up and ran away with the chair to which she had been strapped for the procedure. While his patroness did not permit herself to be operated on, it is clear from Klein's final note why she felt herself to be ugly and wanted to undertake such an operation; such an operation, he notes, should be thought of for those who had actually lost their noses through the pernicious actions of syphilis.

But is not the princess's problem one of the marking of disease and social rejection on her face? Her saddle-nose – whatever its actual cause – is a sign of the owner's disease, indeed a mark of congenital syphilis, and therefore of her ugliness. Ugliness is the result of disease and marks the soul as diseased, as 'unhappy'. And her unhappiness is the evident fact that she is not erotic or attractive. Her illness, that bane of nineteenth-century medicine, hereditary syphilis, is marked on her face. The visibility of inherited syphilis becomes a trope in and of itself from the eighteenth century. It marks the collective, the family, as well as the individual as diseased and, therefore, undesirable of repro- duction. The face and the body of the child of the syphilitic even in the twentieth century, as in an image of a syphilitic cupid from 1905, is so marked (illus. 38). It is not trivial that Klein's patient was a princess – for from the Reformation to the very beginning of the rise of the bourgeoisie, the general assumption was that the nobility was degener- ate and diseased.[15] Just as surely as her nobility (in her fantasy) was written on her face, so too was her disease – and these categories re- inforced one another. The repair of the saddle-nose through the use of gold, which may have a good chemical basis today in the inertness of the metal, points in the early nineteenth century to a sense of class, as does, of course, the use of a pauper as the subject of the princess's human experiment. The princess desired her visibility as a member of

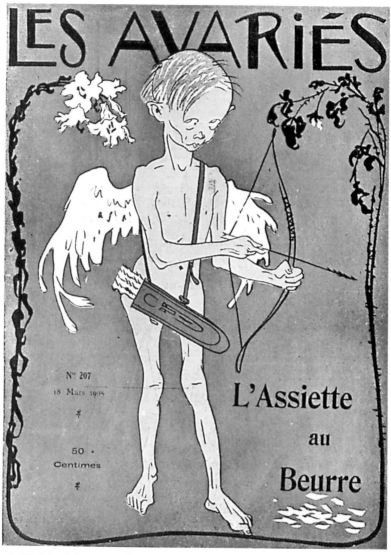

38 *The Injured*, An image of a syphilitic Cupid, from a 1905 issue of the French satirical journal *L'Assiette au Beurre*.

the nobility, without the sexual stigma associated with that group written on her face.

The princess was 'unhappy' because she was seen not only to be ugly, but ugly in a way that indicated her danger toward those about her. The danger of the syphilitic is written on her nose. Even the tiny scar would have marked her face still more. Was the appropriate anxiety about the operation, its potential for pain, infection and scarring, not also an anxiety about being yet further marked and visible?

Thus the nose is coded. A reconstructed nose is as much a visual clue to the diseased nature of the individual as a missing nose or a saddle-nose would be, yet the deformed nose may not be truly a symptom of syphilis or scrofula. The saddle-nose is not necessarily a sign of hereditary syphilis. It can be merely a saddle-nose. What it represents in European culture of the sixteenth to the nineteenth centuries is the link between the destructive powers of sexuality, its expression in sexually transmitted illness, and the absence of the erotic. The very sight of the princess evokes the spectre of disease, and such disease (unlike tuberculosis) cannot be eroticized. This is analogous to stereotypes of certain groups, such as the Irish and the Jew (in different contexts) as being sexual predators, as threatening to pollute society. Here the image of the 'deformed' face of the ethnic group parallels the social anxiety about the sexual. Society's notions of physical deformity are virtually always associated with notions of moral difference.

Thus the ear of the syphilitic is just as marked in such a system as is the nose. Wilhelm Weygandt provided a model of four ears: the 'Darwin-Woolner ear', which marked the degenerate; the paralytic's or syphilitic's ear; 'Wildermuth's ear', which marked the alcoholic; and the idiot's or 'cat's' ear (illus. 39).[16] Each deformation was understood

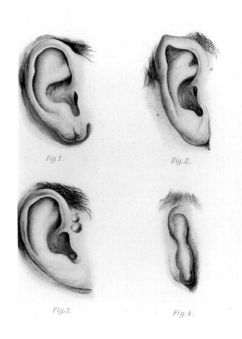

39 The form of the ear reveals character and inheritance. Fig. 1. the primitive ear of the degenerate (the Darwin-Woolner ear); fig. 2. the paralytic's (i.e., syphilitic's) ear; fig. 3. the alcoholic's (Wildermuth's) ear; and fig. 4. the idiot's or 'cat's' ear. From Wilhelm Weygandt's *Atlas und Grundriss der Psychiatrie* (Munich, 1902).

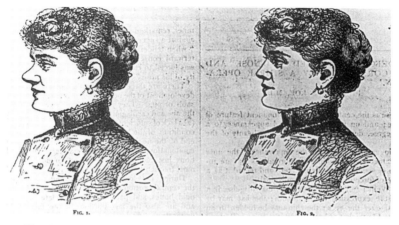

40 The 'before' and 'after' image of the 'pug' nose. From John O. Roe, 'The Deformity Termed "Pug Nose" and its Correction, by a Simple Operation' (*The Medical Record*, 4 June 1887).

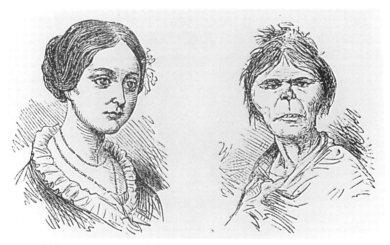

41 The Irish character as revealed in the Irish face: Florence Nightingale vs. Bridget McBruiser. From Samuel R. Wells, *New Physiognomy, or, Signs of Character: As Manifested Through Temperament and External Forms, and Especially in 'The Human Face Divine'* (New York, 1866).

as a sign of some psychological or moral failing. But each sign also represented qualities that were not to be passed on into the collective, as they would weaken or destroy it. And this anxiety about the decay of the collective is also clearly connected to the notion of the anti-erotic.

Different contexts mean the reading of the nose changes and therefore the source of unhappiness also changes. But it remains associated with the diseased and the degenerate through to the close of the nineteenth century. In the 1860s the surgeon John Orlando Roe in Rochester, New York, had developed an operation to 'cure' the 'pug nose' (illus. 40).[17] Based on the profile, Roe divided the image of the nose into five categories: Roman, Greek, Jewish, Snub or Pug, and Celestial. But what is Roe truly curing when he operates on the nose? Roe cites the 'snub-nose' as 'proof of a degeneracy of the human race'. It is a sign of the primitive within, of the atavism of disease – not merely of the individual but of an entire race or nation. In New York State, it was, of course, the Irish profile that was characterized by the snub-nose in the caricatures of the period (illus. 41).[18] Here we have the final internalization of an image of 'ugliness' with all of its cultural associations in the work of a surgeon who can, for the first time, in an age of anaesthesia and antisepsis, truly begin to alter the psyche as he alters the body. The Irish nose is the sign of the anti-erotic, of the sexually dangerous, of the decline into ugliness and decay. It shares a similar space with the nose of the syphilitic as the public sign of the 'ugly' body and therefore the ugly (and dangerous) soul.

The viewer's image of the beautiful, i.e., the erotic, becomes one with his or her own self-image. Paolo Mantegazza in his widely cited *fin de siècle* account of physiognomy stressed that

We, belonging to the higher races, regard as ugly all noses which approach that of the ape, snub, flattened, or very small noses, with nostrils failing in parallelism, and the section of which represents the figure eight. In this respect we even sacrifice the laws of geometry to our atavistic prejudices; we should consider a woman beautiful who had an excessively large nose, rather than pardon a snub one. In Italy we call a large nose aristocratic (especially if it is aquiline), perhaps because the long-nosed conquerors, Greek or Latin, subjugated the autochthonous small-nosed population.[19]

Here it is the long nose of the Italian that is contrasted with the 'ape-like' nose that marked the 'lower' species. This reflects the work, at the close of the eighteenth century, of the Dutch anatomist Petrus Camper, who describes the meaning of the facial angle and its reflex, the nasal index.[20] The nasal index was the line that connected the forehead via the nose to the upper lip; the facial angle was determined by connecting this line with a horizontal line coming from the jaw. This line came to be a means of distinguishing between the human and the other higher anthropoids. Camper's facial angle, which connected all the races of the human race and distinguished all of them from the ape, was also used by many of his contemporaries, such as Theodor Soemmering, and by most of his successors, as the means of creating a hierarchy of the races. Camper himself presents criteria for the beautiful face in his study. Indeed, he defines the 'beautiful face' as one in which the facial line creates an angle of 100° to the horizontal (p. 62). The African is the least beautiful (and therefore the least erotic) because he/she is closest to the ape in physiognomy, went the later reading of Camper.

Camper's work was misused to argue for the identity of the African and the ape as a different species from the European. But it is clear that Camper does provide a very different aesthetics, which reflects the erotic criteria of his day. If for Mantegazza the long nose was the epitome of the attractive, there were different readings of the long nose in Dutch culture: it is the nose of the Jew. The nose of the Jew set the Jew apart as unattractive. And the Jew was virtually as ugly as the African because the Jew's physiognomy was understood to be closer to the African than to the European. Camper also saw the physiognomy of the Jew as immutable:

There is no nation which is as clearly indentifiable as the Jews: men, women, children, even when they are first born, bear the sign of their origin. I have often spoken about this with the famed painter of historical subjects [Benjamin] West, to whom I mentioned my difficulty in capturing the national essence of the Jews. He was of the opinion that this must be sought in the curvature of the nose. I cannot deny that the nose has much to do with this, and that it bears a resemblance to the form of the Mongol (whom I had often observed in London and of which I possess a facial cast), but this is not sufficient for me. For this reason, I feel that the famed painter J[acob] de Wit has painted many men with beards in the Meeting Room of the Inner Council [in Amsterdam] but no Jews (p. 7).

If the Irish nose represented the degenerate in New York State in the 1880s, then the anti-Semitic representation of the Jewish nose – so widely present in the literature of the *fin de siècle* – itself shaped the Jew's response to the Jew's own nose, as I have elsewhere discussed (illus. 42).[21] Thus the French turn of the century anti-Semitic pamphleteer 'Dr Celticus' presents an anatomy of the Jew in which the 'hooked nose' represents the 'true Jew'. 'Nasality' here becomes the foremost visual representation of the 'primitiveness of the Semitic race'.[22]

How could one eliminate the symptom of the 'nostrility' of the Jew, that sign which everyone at the close of the nineteenth century associated with the Jew's visibility? An answer was supplied by Jacques Joseph, a highly acculturated young German-Jewish surgeon in *fin de siècle* Berlin.[23] Born Jakob Joseph, this physician had altered his Jewish name when studying medicine in Berlin and Leipzig. Joseph was a typical acculturated Jew of the period. He had been a member of one of the conservative dueling fraternities and bore the scars of the sabre-

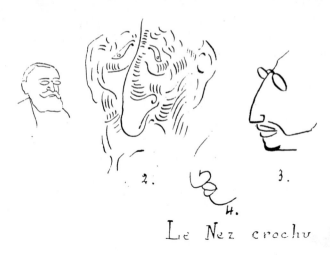

Le Nez crochu

42 The image of the 'hooked' Jewish nose from the anti-Semitic physiological study of the Jew's body by 'Dr Celticus', *Les 19 Tares corporelles visibles pur reconnaître un juif* (Paris, 1903).

dueling with pride. A dueling scar marked the socially healthy individual.

The scarred Jacques Joseph was a trained orthopaedic surgeon who had been the assistant of Julius Wolff, one of the leaders in that field. Among Wolff's most important findings was the 'law of the transformation of the skeleton', which argued that every function of the skeleton could be described through the laws of mechanics, and that any change of the relationship between single components of the skeleton would lead to a functional and physiological change in the external form of the entire body.[24] Wolff's major contribution to the treatment of diseases of the leg was his development of a therapeutic procedure by which a club foot could be corrected through the use of a specialized dressing that altered the very shape of the foot.[25] Orthopaedics, more than any other medical specialty of the period, presented the challenge of altering the visible errors of development so as to restore a 'normal' function. Wolff's approach also stressed the interrelationship between all aspects of the body. Among his procedures was corrective surgery as well as the use of appliances. Joseph's interests did not lie with the foot, another sign of Jewish inferiority, but elsewhere in the anatomy.

In 1896 Joseph had undertaken a corrective procedure on a child with protruding ears, which, while successful, caused him to be dismissed from Wolff's clinic. This was cosmetic, not reconstructive,

85

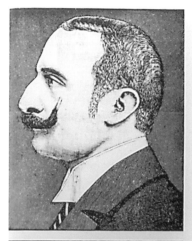

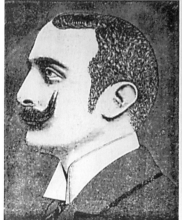

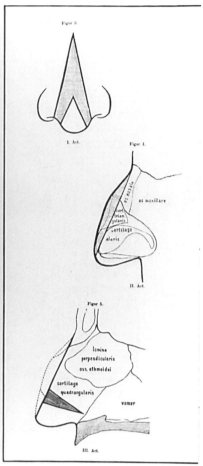

43 'Before' and 'after' images of the first modern rhinoplasty and the procedure itself. From Jacques Joseph, 'Über die operative Verkleinerung einer Nase (Rhinimiosis)', *Berliner klinische Wochenschrift* XL (1898).

surgery.[26] One simply did not undertake surgical procedures for vanity's sake, he was told. This was not a functional disability, such as a club foot. The child was not suffering from any physical ailment that could be cured through surgery. Here reconstructive surgery became aesthetic surgery.

Joseph opened a private surgical practice in Berlin. In January 1898 a 28-year-old man came to him, having heard of the successful operation on the child's ears (illus. 43). The man complained that 'his nose was the source of considerable annoyance. Wherever he went, everybody stared at him; often, he was the target of remarks or ridiculing gestures. On account of this he became melancholic,

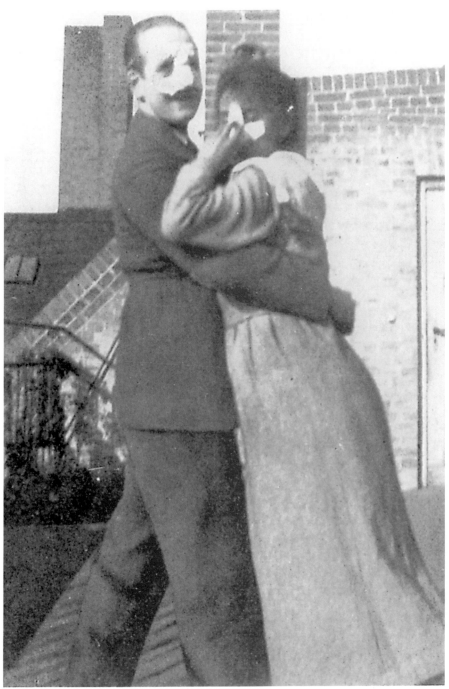

44 Jacques Joseph supplied images of his happy patients in his comprehensive textbook of rhinoplasty. From his *Nasenplastik und sonstige Gesichtsplastik* (Leipzig, 1931).

withdrew almost completely from social life, and had the earnest desire to be relieved of this deformity.'[27] Joseph took the young man's case and proceeded to perform the first modern cosmetic rhinoplasty. On 11 May 1898 he reported on this operation before the Berlin Medical Society. In that report Joseph provided a 'scientific' rationale for performing a medical procedure on what was an otherwise completely healthy individual: 'the psychological effect of the operation is of utmost importance. The depressed attitude of the patient subsided completely. He is happy to move around unnoticed [illus. 44]. His happiness in life has increased, his wife was glad to report; the patient who formerly avoided social contact now wishes to attend and give parties. In other words, he is happy over the results' (p. 180). The patient no longer felt himself marked by the form of his nose. He was cured of his 'disease', which was his visibility. Joseph had undertaken a surgical procedure that had cured his patient's psychological disorder! (It is not an accident that psychoanalysis was being developed at precisely the same time by two Jewish neurologists in Vienna as cosmetic surgery began in the clinic of two Jewish orthopaedists of Berlin. Both were modes of curing the psyche of illnesses that manifested themselves in the racially marked body, and both were concerned with the nose as the visible site of these illnesses.)

Joseph's task was to cure the psyche of his patients by making them 'beautiful', and the result, for him, was happy patients.[28] When he sought out models for what body would make his patients happy and, therefore, healthy, he turned to classical models of the body similar to those used by Ernst Brücke, whose work I discussed in the previous chapter. Joseph went to Dürer for his mathematical formulae of beauty and deformity. The beautiful is the regular and the proportioned. Whether the nose or the breast, balance and proportion are the hallmarks of the beautiful, and therefore healthy, body. His ideal female face has a 'greco-roman profile with a 33° facial angle'. What is striking is that his choice of an image is a portrait of his (Jewish) wife. His 'proof' for her beauty is a drawing he reproduces by Leonardo da Vinci (illus. 45, 46). The norms for Joseph's ideal of beauty are taken from high art, with all the status high art had for the educated German of the time. Joseph's wife is beautiful because she resembles a work of high art. And this becomes his and his patient's ideal of the healthy. Jews who do not look like the aesthetic norms of European artistic 'beauty' are thus sick.

Like his first patient, Joseph's subsequent patients are so glad about their new (even unveiled) status that they dance with joy! And Joseph reproduces images of their 'spontaneous' dancing in his textbook of

45 The ideal female profile actualized, 'with Greek and Roman qualities; an unretouched image'. Actually a photograph of Jacques Joseph's wife, from his *Nasenplastik und sonstige Gesichtsplastik*.

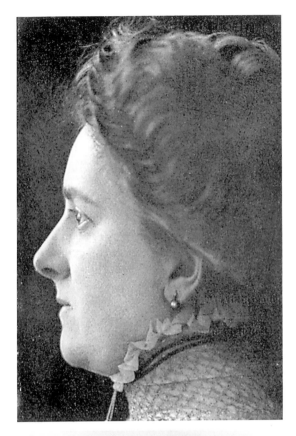

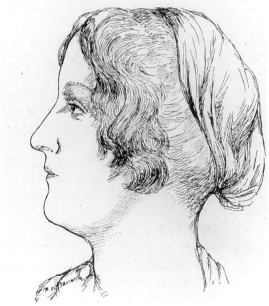

46 'The ideal female profile', after a sketch by Leonardo da Vinci. From Jacques Joseph's *Nasenplastik und sonstige Gesichtsplastik*.

cosmetic surgery as proof of their psychic cure. For it is the ill mind that is the result of the 'misshapen' body. Joseph's patients have become beautiful people, for the blemish on their character, their racial identity, is no longer written on their visages. They, like Joseph's first patient, become newly eroticized and sexualized.

The link, between being seen as different and being unerotic haunts the late nineteenth-century literature on cosmetic surgery. The stigma of the missing nose has now been attached to the Semitic (or the Irish) nose. Paul Schilder, one of Freud's colleagues at the University of Vienna, later went to New York University, where in 1935 he revised and expanded his views of body imagery in his study *The Image and Appearance of the Human Body*, a book that details the complex interaction between the realities of the body, the perception of the self and the representation of the self within culture. Never before nor since has there been as complex a rationale for aesthetic surgery.[29] Schilder recounted the case of A.M., a 29-year-old male whose complaint was that he was 'too ugly and that no girl who was in any way attractive ever fell in love with him'. His 'nose was particularly offensive to him since it was in his opinion too Jewish' (p. 258). He associated this with 'his father's family because of their very Semitic appearance and specific Jewish qualities'. Appearance became associated for Schilder's patient with a specific negative disposition, and this in turn with his own ugliness and his sexual rejection by a young woman. Jewishness sensed on the body becomes converted into ugliness of the spirit. As a result he undertook to have his nose reshaped. Schilder's analysis with A.M. revealed that the 'nose' – following Freud's earlier view – represented the family of his father whose 'Semitic' features and resultant character marked him in his fantasy. In the course of his analysis Schilder tied the anxiety about the father within to the analysand's own sense of the inferiority of his own body. Schilder evokes the classic model of castration anxiety, noting that the patient 'when he was young saw his father's sex organ which seemed too big to him. A few years later the thought came to him that his own organ was too small'. Thus the analysand came to see 'beauty only in the body of others and [he] missed it in his own body'. His drive for an aesthetic in his self was limited by the sense of the inferiority of his body – of the presence in his internalized sense of himself of the body of the father, and the symbol of the father's body was the nose. But all of this is to be understood in the light of the social context of reading the patient's sense of his own body. 'Beauty and ugliness', writes Schilder, are certainly in the single individual, but are social phenomena of the utmost importance. They regulate the sex activities in human relations, and not only in the manifest heterosexual activities, but also the homosexual ones which are so important for the social structure. In the case of our patient, the admiration for his friends who were, in his opinion, better endowed than himself, plays an enormous part. Our own body-image and the body-image of others, their beauty and ugliness, thus becomes the basis for our sexual and social activities. We like to believe that our standards of beauty are absolute (p. 268).

Schilder sees the patient only after his rhinoplasty. The patient 'quoted others who said that before his operation his face was more character-istic [read Jewish] than it was now, but seemed on the whole rather contented with the result'. This patient eventually breaks with his religious identity and converts to Catholicism, the ultimate form of invisibility in Catholic Vienna.

Heightened anti-Semitic pressure in no way mitigates the notion that the permanence of the Jew's face marked the inherent difference between the Jew and the Aryan. The German-Jewish poet George Mannheimer, writing in exile in Prague in 1937, could evoke the 'strange face' of the Jew:

> I know, you don't love us.
> We are not like the others.
> People who rest and people who wander
> Have a totally different face.

> I know, you don't love us.
> We have swum through too many streams.
> But, let us come to rest,
> Then we shall have the same face.[30]

Mannheimer's text evokes the potential elimination of any 'ugliness' associated with the 'nomadic' nature ascribed to the Jew. Here it is not surgical intervention but acculturation that will alter the internalized sense of alienation marking the face of the Jew.

Here we can evoke Jean-Jacques Rousseau, who commented in his novel of education, *Émile* (1762), that 'the way in which the Author of our being has shaped our heads does not suit us; we must have them modelled from without by midwives and from within by philoso-phers'.[31] For Joseph articulated the basic premise of modern aesthetic surgery, that the correction of perceived physical anomalies (not pathologies) was a means of repairing not the body but the psyche. And this at exactly the same moment in modern history that Freud had begun to understand the basis for his own approach to curing the hysterical body, with all its physical signs and symptoms, through the treatment of the psyche! Aesthetic surgery comes to be understood as 'organopsychic therapy', in which 'it is exclusively the altered or defective form of the pathologically and anatomically normal organ that causes psychic conflicts'.[32] We see at the close of the nineteenth century a 'modelling from within' by surgeons rather than by philosophers, but surgeons whose role is to cure not the body but the psyche.

Sexuality and the aesthetic are closely linked to the question of the beautiful, the truly healthy. While there are some limitations to the notion of the beautiful (there is the image of the beautiful as trap), in general our desire is to limit the diseased to the world of the ugly. The ugly is anti-erotic rather than merely unaesthetic. It is denied the ability to reproduce.

5 Mark Twain and Hysteria in the Holy Land

Twain's World

The equation of beauty with health and ugliness with illness is fundamental in the Western understanding of the body. Its powerful racist potential has permeated the works of even the most 'liberal' writers and thinkers. Racial differences were understood as differences in character, even in the character of the physician. William Osler, one of the pre-eminent physicians of the early twentieth century, signalled this in his 'Israel and Medicine' (1914):

> In estimating the position of Israel in the human values we must remember that the quest for righteousness is oriental, the quest for knowledge occidental. With the great prophets of the East – Moses, Isaiah, Mahomet – the word was 'Thus saith the Lord'; with the great seers of the West, from Thales and Aristotle to Archimedes and Lucretius, it was 'What says Nature?' They illustrate two opposite views of man and his destiny – in the one he is an 'angelus sepultus' in a muddy vesture of decay; in the other, he is the 'young light-hearted master' of the world, in it to know it, and by knowing to conquer.[1]

For Osler, medicine, and perhaps even health, is Greek, not Jewish. The association of healing and race was a commonplace at the turn of the century. It certainly plays an interesting role in the works of the American writer most widely read at the *fin de siècle*, Mark Twain.

There has been increased interest recently in Mark Twain's essay 'Concerning the Jews', which appeared in the September 1898 issue of *Harper's Magazine*.[2] Indeed, there has even been speculation that Freud's last public statement on the nature of anti-Semitism was a paraphrase of Twain's work.[3] Twain's essay responded to a reader's enquiry following his ironic account in the August issue of the anti-Semitic rhetoric of the 'debate' in the Austrian parliament concerning the bill mandating Czech as the official language of Bohemia. Twain's reasoned answer, along with the addendum concerning the role of the Jew as soldier, make up one of the most complex documents written against anti-Semitism in late nineteenth-century America. Yet it reveals presuppositions about the special nature of the Jew noted even by Twain's contemporaries, such as M. S. Levy, who wrote in 1899 that 'from the many statements Mark Twain makes regarding the various traits of the Jews, it is plain that they are not only tinged with malice and prejudice, but are incorrect and false'.[4] It is clear that Twain's intent in writing his essay 'concerning the Jews' was to counter the growing anti-Semitism that accompanied the increase in East European Jewish immigration to the United States. Twain's shifting, sometimes contradictory, positions concerning the Jews were acknowledged by his contemporaries. What is important, and has not been noted by the critics, either contemporary or contemporaneous, is that Twain shifts the underlying rhetoric of his argument from one which sees the nature of the Jews as immutable to one which understands it as socially constructed. Here I will examine three interrelated questions: the image of the Jew in Twain's earliest writing and its affinity to the model of the 'diseased Jew'; the various racial models of the diseased Jew that existed in European and American thought throughout the nineteenth century; and the continuity or discontinuity of Twain's later views with his earlier ones. First we must comprehend that there was an earlier, as yet unread, image of the Jew in Twain's work published decades before the more widely cited essay 'Concerning the Jews'.

I will thus not begin with this late, 'liberal' essay (though I shall refer to it later in this analysis), but with Twain's first extended representation of the Jews in his most popular book, *The Innocents Abroad, or The New Pilgrim's Progress*.[5] What I shall be examining is its representation of illness and the relationship of this model to contemporary discussions of Jewish illnesses. This travel account, first published in 1869, reflects a specific debate about the Jew's body that occurred during Reconstruction. This is part of a larger debate of the time on the inheritability of identity. *The Innocents Abroad* recounts Twain's journey to Europe and the Holy Land during 1867. One of its central themes is the traveller's experience of disease. Disease is a concept closely linked to religion and the exotic. This theme quickly becomes one of the structuring principles of the philosophy of history that underlies Twain's account: he and his friends move backward in time as they travel eastward in space. And, as we shall see, no people is more ancient, or remote, or diseased than the Jews. For Twain, the tracing of disease becomes a commentary on the role of the Jews in Western civilization. Such underlying views would seem to run counter to the stated intentions of Twain's essay of 1898.

The Innocents Abroad begins with the reprinting of the announcement for the tour. This list of particulars included in the advantages of the ship, the *Quaker City*, the fact that 'an experienced physician will be on board' (p. 18). The advertisement of such a provision was not accidental. Disease and death were understood to be ubiquitous in exotic locales. The American travellers experience disease and death in the exotic locales they visit in Europe and the Middle East. This in turn defines the Americans as the curable, if not the healthy, and a 'white' United States as a place where there may be illness, but where there is also modern 'scientific' medicine and the potential for remedy. (Twain, as we shall see, assumes that the Native American is predisposed to illness.) For, even with all of the minor illnesses that the American travellers suffer, there is no parallel in their experience to the ever-mounting horrors they see on their trip. Medicine is on their side, as is an unqualified belief in that science. It is the reality of disease and death that haunts Twain's representation of his travels eastward.

Earlier American travellers on the Grand Tour had recounted their own fascination with the spectre of disease, but always within the frame of the aesthetic. Among the standard stops on the Grand Tour were the exhibitions of anatomical figures in the museums of Bologna, Florence, Rome and Vienna.[6] Florence especially, and specifically the 'Royal and Imperial Museum of Physics and Natural History' (called 'La Specola' because of its observatory), founded in 1775, became the mecca for travellers fascinated by the world of decay. Represented in the collection at Florence were a number of the great masters of wax-casting, especially the famed Sicilian wax-modeller Gaetano Giulo Zummo. These sculptors were responsible for many of the anatomical exhibitions and much of the religious art in this medium throughout Italy and France. The traveller experienced these genres as one where the anatomized body and the body of the martyred saint were represented by the same aesthetic devices.

These collections of anatomical art became a focus for the visits of Americans on the Grand Tour. They were offered a sense of the Sublime, the most overwhelming sensation to be had within nature. This was nature frozen in the form of the wax cast, rather than in the stinking cadavers of the anatomical theatre. Henry Wadsworth Long-fellow saw these figures on his tour of the Continent in the 1830s, and sensed both their reality and the unreality that one must ascribe to the medium of the wax sculpture:

Zumbo [sic] . . . must have been a man of the most gloomy and saturnine imagination, and more akin to the worm than most of us, thus to have reveled night and day in the hideous mysteries of death, corruption, and the charnel house. It is strange how this representation haunts one. It is like a dream of the sepulcher, with its loathsome corpses, with 'the blackening, the swelling, the bursting of the trunk – the worm, the rat, and the tarantula at work.' You breathe more freely as you step out into the bright sunshine and the crowded, busy streets next meet your eye, you are ready to ask, Is this indeed a representation of reality?[7]

The dream of the real, or perhaps the nightmare of death, of the body corrupt, of the body putrefied, is 'real' only because it tricks the highest sense, sight; it is 'unreal', a false representation because it lacks the other senses. Real putrefaction would not only be dynamic, it would swarm with flies, and it would stink. Longfellow's vision was of the permanence of corruption, of the immutability of mutability, all images so contradictory that they lead to a questioning of the very body itself. Longfellow saw all this in the work of art representing death and decay.

The world of exotic religion that these American travellers experienced was also closely associated in the wax cast with the erotic and with death. As late as 1858, Nathaniel Hawthorne (on his Grand Tour) sensed the proximity of these associations: 'And here, within a glass case, there is the representation of an undraped little boy in wax, very prettily modelled, and holding up a heart that looks like a bit of red sealing-wax. If I had found him anywhere else, I should have taken him for Cupid; but being in an oratory, I presume him to have some religious signification.'[8]

Perhaps because of Twain's frontier exposure to public images of disease and physical corruption, he was fascinated less with this type of aesthetized corpse than with the dreary realities of European daily life. For Twain, it is not the image of decay and the body which fascinates, but the dead and decaying body itself.

In Paris, one of their early stops in Europe, Twain's travellers in *The Innocents Abroad* first visit Notre Dame, where they are shown relics similar to Hawthorne's little wax figure. But here they include the 'bloody robe' of the Archbishop of Paris assassinated on the Parisian barricades in 1848 as well as 'the bullet that killed him, and the two vertebrae in which it was lodged' (p. 105). Twain's comment that 'these people have a somewhat singular taste to the matter of relics' links (as do the comments of Longfellow and Hawthorne) the representation of the body within the rituals of Christianity (here, especially Catholicism) and the barbarous dismemberment and display of the body (illus. 47). Little surprise that after the Cathedral, the travellers' next stop is 'the Morgue, that horrible receptacle for the dead who die mysteriously and leave the manner of their taking off a dismal secret' (p. 105). There they see the body of a drowned man 'naked, swollen, purple', gawked at by the passers by, 'people, I thought, who live upon strong excitements, and who attend the exhibitions of the Morgue regularly, just as other people go to see theatrical spectacles every night. When one of these

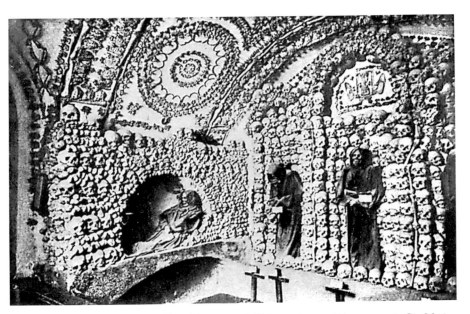

47 'A corner in the Capuchin convent': Using an image of the ossuary in Sta Maria della Concezione, Rome, in the illustrated edition of his *Innocents Abroad* (New York, 1899), Mark Twain moves the close relationship between the idea of death and organized religion ever more southward.
The following three plates are also taken from the illustrated edition that was approved by Twain.

looked in and passed on, I could not help thinking: "Now this don't afford you any satisfaction – a party with his head shot *off* is what you need"' (p. 106). Such a body would have been the body of the Archbishop of Paris as exposed in the Cathedral of Notre Dame. Twain has established the relationship between religion, especially exotic religions such as Catholicism, and the dead or dying body (illus. 48).[9]

The link between disease and the exotic increases as Twain travels East. On entering Constantinople he is reminded of the 'dwarfs' and 'cripples' he had seen on the streets of Genoa, Milan and Naples. His Italian experience was nothing compared to the 'very heart and home of cripples and human monsters' that is Constantinople. There Twain sees in the very flesh the deformed and mutilated – a woman with three legs, two of them withered; a man with an eye in his cheek. The normally mutilated, 'a mere damaged soldier of crutches would never make a cent. It would pay him to get a piece of his head taken off, and cultivate a wen like a carpet sack' (p. 285). All these horrors of the flesh are seen by the travellers on their way to the mosque of St Sophia. The association of disease and religion is increasing exponentially. For in

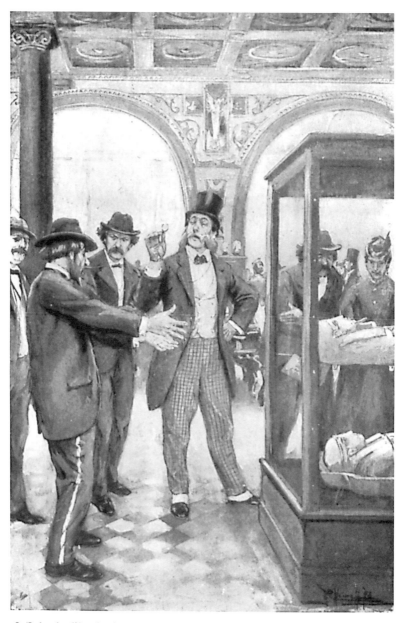

48 'Is he dead?' – the American tourists find themselves in confronting an exhibition of mummies. A plate from Twain's *Innocents Abroad*.

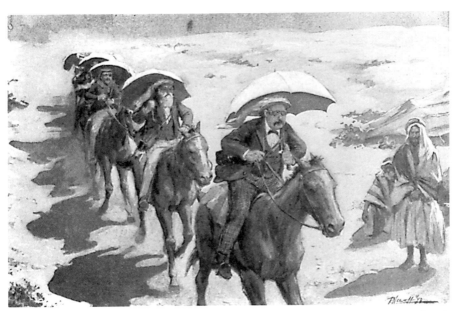

49 'Our party of Eight' enter the Holy Land. A plate from Twain's *Innocents Abroad*.

Paris Twain had to link two isolated places in the city in order to link religion and disease; in Constantinople disease, deformity and dirt are everywhere, invading, indeed defining, the very presence of the mosque itself (p. 286).

The closer Twain and his party get to the Holy Land, the stronger the link. In Damascus – on their way to the Holy Land – the very sight of the city causes Twain to begin to quote for the first time from what is his (and his companions') true guidebook on this journey, the Bible (illus. 49). For the travels of the innocents in Twain's account are a disguised account of a pilgrim's progress, but the progress of a pilgrim already doubting the veracity of his own faith. The sight of Damascus evokes Paul's sojourn there and the origins of Pauline Christianity, 'that bold missionary career which he prosecuted 'til his death' (p. 365). Twain's own ambivalence toward religion in general takes on the coloration of his anxiety about the link between disease, death and belief. Twain does not see this decay and disease as taking part in isolation or at a distance from himself. Rather, he slowly comes to understand that his own cultural perspective is itself a product of a religious world view, and that world view is that of the Jews. It is therefore not the New Testament by which Twain comprehends the Holy Land.

The image Twain uses to close this chapter and to introduce us to the Holy Land is not taken from the New Testament, but from the Old.

He quotes Naaman's words from 2 Kings 5, who praised the waters of Damascus as 'better than all the waters of Israel. May I not wash in them and be clean?' For Naaman, 'the favorite of the king', was a leper, and his house in Damascus had been turned into a leper hospital, whose 'inmates expose their horrid deformities and hold up their hands and beg for buckseesh when a stranger enters' (p. 367). Twain's response is one of horror: 'One cannot appreciate the horror of this disease until he looks upon it in all its ghastliness, in Naaman's ancient dwelling in Damascus. Bones all twisted out of shape, great knots protruding from face and body, joints decaying and dropping away – horrible!' (p. 367). To this point Twain had stayed distant from the horrors of death. Death was the business of others – the visitors to Notre Dame or the Rue Morgue, or those unfortunates who exposed their mutilations in Catholic Italy or Muslim Turkey. In Damascus, however, Twain immediately internalizes the horrors he sees. It is in Damascus, the city of Naaman the Leper, that Twain is struck ill (illus. 50).

Twain spent his final day in Damascus after visiting the leper hospital, suffering from 'cholera, or cholera morbus' (p. 368). Given his symptoms, it is clear that his intestinal complaint is what we today would call 'turista' or, perhaps, Naaman's Revenge, or what was then called 'cholera morbus'. It was hardly cholera as understood in the late nineteenth century.[10] His response to his symptoms was hysterically to apostrophize his healthy, American audience – as if his stomach cramps were the sign of his own corrupt nature. His association of the world he has entered with disease has now infiltrated his very being, his inner sense of self. Twain comes to realize that the association of death, illness and religion is not merely the fancy of exotic practices (Catholicism) or religions (Islam) or of spaces that are unrelated to his sense of self (Paris, Naples, Constantinople). Now he has to struggle with the fact that this association belongs to his world, the world of backwoods Christianity represented by The Book that formed his sense of self, the Bible. But Damascus, the gateway to the world of the Bible, in contrast to the diseased nature of the Holy Land, retrospectively becomes his 'one pleasant reminiscence of this Palestine excursion'.[11] The loathing Twain comes to feel for the diseased world of the Bible confuses his text. The hysterical discovery that the disease he had attributed to others is part of him creates physical symptoms, revulsion and nausea. Nausea in this text unites the diseased ancient past from which Twain had thought he was so distant, and his antiseptic present. What was external to Twain and confined to Constantinople, Twain has now internalized as a symbolic represen-

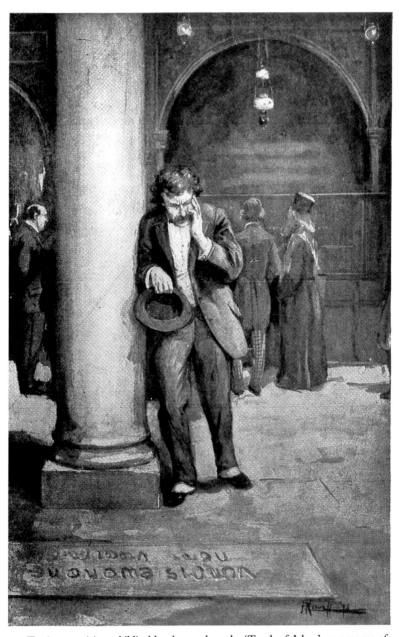

50 Twain uses visits to biblical locales, such as the 'Tomb of Adam', as a means of stressing the comic aspect of the world of the Jews. Jewish tradition places Adam's grave at Hebron, where Twain's party visits it; Christian tradition places it at Calvary, in order that the blood of the second Adam (Christ) was able to pour over the head of the first. A plate from Twain's *Innocents Abroad*.

tation of the means by which he belongs to this world. Illness is real, it exists in the very fabric of the world around him, and it infiltrates even his being. Illness is tied closely to religious belief, to 'superstition', which the ironic Twain and his appreciative reader must see as remote from themselves. In this frame of mind, Twain sets off for the Holy Land. The very first experience he has 'just stepping over the border and entering into the long-sought Holy Land' (p. 372) is disease.

On 17 September 1867 Twain entered the Holy Land with seven companions. There he finds that the very ground on which the Saviour walked, 'that Jesus looked on in the flesh' (p. 373), is the land of disease.[12] 'Standing on ground that was once actually pressed by the feet of the Saviour', Twain sees himself surrounded by 'the usual assemblage of squalid humanity', which in its passive suffering reminds him of the Native Americans: 'They remind me much of Indians, did these people. . . . They sat in silence, and with tireless patience watched our every motion with that vile, uncomplaining impoliteness which is so truly Indian, and which makes a white man so nervous and uncomfortable and savage that he wants to exterminate the whole tribe. These people about us had other peculiarities, which I have noticed in the noble red man, too: they were infested with vermin, and the dirt caked on them till it amounted to bark' (pp. 374–5). The children are covered with flies, they suffer from sore eyes which eventually lead to blindness in many of them. And in their passivity and acceptance of illness they are the very antithesis of the white American: 'And, would you suppose that an American mother could sit for an hour, with her child in her arms, and let a hundred flies roost upon its eyes all that time undisturbed? I see that every day' (p. 375). Twain's 'sight' is a mark of his American health, as opposed to the blindness of the inhabitants of the Holy Land.

Once the waiting multitudes learn that among the travellers is a physician, Dr J. B. Birch of Hannibal, Missouri, they come in droves. Are they not attracted by exactly that same faith which moved the steamship line back in the United States to advertise so prominently the presence of a physician on board the *Quaker City*? 'The lame, the halt, the blind, the leprous – all the distempers that are bred of indolence, dirt, and iniquity – were represented' (p. 375). And the doctor ministered to them with his 'dread, mysterious power' and 'phials . . . of white powder'. For these diseased individuals 'he was gifted like a god' (p. 376). The physician as 'god' is a mirror of one of the central metaphors of Christianity, that of Christ as physician: 'and great multitudes came together to hear, and to be healed by him of their infirmities' (Luke 4:15).

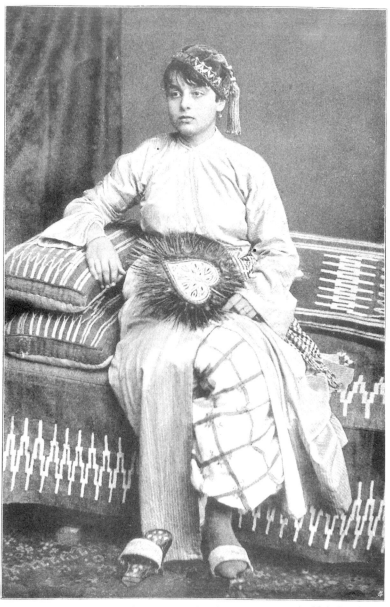

51 In contrast to Twain, with his image of the Jewish woman in the Holy Land, Jewish savants of the late 19th century sought to present the women there as idealized countertypes to the image of the East European Jewish woman. Here a 'Jewish woman in Palestine' from Carl Heinrich Stratz, *Was sind Juden? Eine ethnographisch-anthropologische Studie* (Vienna, 1903).

And here Twain plays the card he had been holding from the moment he and his companions left the United States. For it is the very despair of these individuals that makes the very wonders of the historical Christ comprehensible, a factor understood in the abstract in Western religion but written on the very skin of the inhabitants of the Holy Land:

Christ knew how to preach to these simple, superstitious, disease-tortured creatures: He healed the sick. They flock to our poor human doctor this morning when the fame of what he had done to the sick child went abroad through the land. . . . The ancestors of these – people precisely like them in color, dress, manners, customs, simplicity – flocked in vast multitudes after Christ, and when they saw him make the afflicted whole with a word, it was no wonder that they worshipped Him. No wonder his deeds were the talk of the nation. No wonder the multitude that followed Him was so great that at one time – thirty miles from here – they had to let a sick man down through the roof because no approach could be made to the door; no wonder His audiences were so great at Galilee that he had to preach from a ship removed a little distance from the shore; no wonder that even in the desert places about Bethsaida, five thousand invaded His solitude, and He had to feed them by a miracle or else see them suffer for their confiding faith and devotion; no wonder when there was a great commotion in a city in those days, one neighbor explained it to another in words to this effect; 'They say that Jesus of Nazareth is come!' (p. 376).

Here is the secret of Christ's historical mission – he cured the diseased in a world tormented by infirmity. His miracles mirrored the needs of the world in which he found himself. But his audience was persuaded only by the reality of their experience of their own disease. They were materialists who could only understand the transcendental (if transcendental he was) if it were internalized and written on their skins.

But Twain's mid-nineteenth-century Palestinian Arabs (he does not say whether Moslem or Christian) were not biblical Jews. He stresses the fact that he is speaking in the present about the Arabs of the Holy Land, for one of the children treated by his travelling companion, the physician, is the daughter of the local sheik (illus. 51). Nevertheless Twain sees 'this poor, ragged handful of sores and sin' now inhabiting the Holy Land as identical in all respects with the Jews who dwelt there at the time of Jesus (p. 377). Their physiognomy is unchanged and this is also reflected in the unchanged nature of their diseased bodies. Christ preached to the biblical Jews whose sorry physical state made them believe in him. The most efficacious way of persuading them of his mission was to cure them of their afflictions. But the Jews remain essentially uncured, as they remain unconverted to Christianity. The 'blindness' that afflicts the inhabitants of the Holy Land is both an

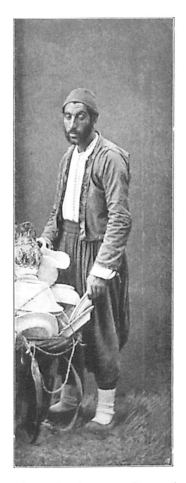

52 Twain imagined his Egyptians as 'Orientals' just as he imagined the Jews. Here an 'Islamic merchant' from Stratz's *Was sind Juden.*

explanation of a perceived reality (the relationship between flies and blindness) as well as proof of the health that emanates from the American and is represented by Twain's Christian insight. This is the central Christian trope about the nature of the Jew, for those who 'lacketh . . . [knowledge of our Lord Jesus Christ are] blind, and cannot see afar off, and hath forgotten that he was purged from his old sins' (2 Peter 1:8–9). For it is 'that blindness in part is happened to Israel, until the fulness of the Gentiles be come in' (Romans 11:25). Jews are blind; Christians see.

For Twain, the image of Jesus is linked to his ability to heal. He ironically imagines the young Jesus in these terms: 'Recall infant Christ's pranks on his school-mates – striking boys dead – withering their hands.'[13] Jesus as a child does precisely what the adult Jesus undoes – he strikes his playmates with illness and death. One can think of the account of the first Jews Twain ever saw in Hannibal, the Levin boys, and the 'shudder' that went through all of the other boys in town as they discussed whether they should crucify the Levin boys.[14] Jews were automatically associated with the act of crucifixion and were seen as literally defiling the Christian world by their presence. But for Twain these Jews 'were clothed in the damp and cobwebby mold of antiquity. They carried me back to Egypt, and in imagination I moved among the Pharaohs . . .' (illus. 52).[15] The present evoked the past. In 1853 Twain could still speak of Jews 'desecrating' two historical houses in Philadelphia.[16] This image of pollution is closely linked in the world of the Jews. Twain can and does draw a clear distinction between the Jews and himself – they are corrupt and he (and all the other Protestant Christians) are the antithesis. And yet on entering the Holy Land, the inescapable fact, hitherto understood in the abstract, but here suddenly writ large for even Twain to see, was that all of those beloved figures of the Old and the New Testament were Jews – Jesus as well as Naaman. But they were Jews like the present-day inhabitants of the Holy Land. They were diseased just like Twain himself in Damascus. Twain needs to separate his Christian-American identity from the image of the Jew that was part of his cultural inheritance. Everyone (including Mark Twain) has the potential to become ill, but the Jews are illness incarnate.

Twain presents the Jews as the sum of their diseased nature and its reflection of their essence, reaching from the biblical leper Naaman to their contemporary surrogates. It mirrors Twain's own questioning of his internalization of the Judaeo-Christian presuppositions of the Bible. Why does Christ appear to the multitudes? It is only to cure and thus answer the needs of the Jews. Disease and religion are linked, but they are linked in the essence of the Jew. The racial identity of the Jew is unchanged across centuries, even though the religious identity of the inhabitants of the Holy Land may have shifted. Twain reads this not merely as a reflex of the space in which the Jews are located. There is a *fin de siècle* school of thought, best represented by the German anthropologist Friedrich Ratzel, which argued that the nature of a race is a reflex of the geographical space in which it is found.[17] The nature of the Jews is tied to the space they 'naturally' inhabit. For Twain the movement into the Holy Land is also a movement back in time; the world has shaped the peoples found in it, and this is now reflected (by the process of a Lamarckian inheritance) in their inherent nature. The nature of the Jews is tied not only to their space but also to their historical times. It is the illusion of a permanent space that forms the Jews and their 'essence' as a diseased people. The Arabs of the Holy Land are merely unchanged biblical Jews in disguise. Jewish immutability is a commonplace of late nineteenth-century anthropological and medical science. In Richard Andree's 1881 study of Jewish folklore the central question is the relationship between who the Jews are and what their bodies mean. Andree's discussion centres on the permanence of the Jewish racial type, but, more importantly, on its implications. He observed, concerning the conservative nature of the Jewish body and soul:

No other race but the Jews can be traced with such certainty backward for thousands of years, and no other race displays such a constancy of form, none resisted to such an extent the effects of time, as the Jews. Even when he adopts the language, dress, habits, and customs of the people among whom he lives, he still remains everywhere the same. All he adopts is but a cloak, under which the eternal Hebrew survives; he is the same in his facial features, in the structure of his body, his temperament, his character.[18]

And it is the body of the Jew that is the sign of this immutability, and, in the discourse of the late nineteenth century, of his immutable relationship to disease, pathology and death. Twain is responding to a debate about the diseased nature of the Jews that had long been part of Western culture but took an especially striking turn in the latter half of the nineteenth century.

Jews are Diseased

The signs of disease had long marked the Jews as different. The earliest modern Christian images evoked their decrepitude as an aspect of their essence. It was seen as the physical sign of their culpability for the Crucifixion. Johannes Buxtorf, in an account of Jewish beliefs and practices written in 1643 for a fearful Christian audience, catalogued their diseases: epilepsy, the plague, leprosy.[19] Johann Jakob Schudt, the late seventeenth-century Orientalist who was *the* authority on the nature of the difference of the Jews for his time, cited their physical form as diseased and repellent:

Among several hundred of their kind he had not encountered a single person without a blemish or other repulsive feature: for they are either pale and yellow or swarthy; they have in general big heads, big mouths, everted lips, protruding eyes and bristle-like eyelashes, large ears, crooked feet, hands that hang below their knees, and big shapeless warts, or are otherwise asymmetrical and malproportioned in their limbs.[20]

Schudt saw the Jews' diseases as a reflex of their 'Jewishness', of their stubborn refusal to acknowledge the truth of Christianity. What is striking about Schudt's early comment is his seeing the diseased Jew as 'swarthy' in his illness.

How intensively this image of the black Jew haunts the imagination of European society can be seen in a description by the 'liberal' Bavarian writer Johann Pezzl, who travelled to Vienna in the 1780s and described the typical Viennese Jew of his time:

There are about five hundred Jews in Vienna. Their sole and eternal occupation is to counterfeit (*Mauscheln*), salvage, trade in coins, and cheat Christians, Turks, heathens, indeed themselves. . . . This is only the beggarly filth from Canaan which can only be exceeded in filth, uncleanliness, stench, disgust, poverty, dishonesty, pushiness and other things by the trash of the twelve tribes from Galicia. Excluding the Indian fakirs, there is no category of supposed human beings which comes closer to the Orang-Utan than does a Polish Jew. . . . Covered from foot to head in filth, dirt and rags, covered in a type of black sack . . . their necks exposed, the color of a Black, their faces covered up to the eyes with a beard, which would have given the High Priest in the Temple chills, the hair turned and knotted as if they all suffered from the *plica polonica*.[21]

The image of the Viennese Jew is of the Eastern Jew, suffering from the diseases of the East, such as the *Judenkratze*, the fabled skin and hair disease also attributed to the Poles under the designation of the *plica polonica*.[22] The Jews' disease is written on the skin. It is the appearance, the skin-colour, the external manifestations of the Jew that marks the Jew as different. Here Pezzl argues by analogy – the Jews are like the Blacks. When this tradition is transferred into American culture during Reconstruction, the analogy between the Jew and the Black has an even greater salience. For if the Jews are taken to be the same as Blacks, how does the Christian white reader, especially the Christian white physician, relate to the marked nature of the Jew's body? This complex American tradition of reading the Jew's body is where *The Innocents Abroad, or The New Pilgrims' Progress* can best be placed.

The very charge that the Jews had a diseased nature – whether because of their essence or because of their experience – was hotly debated in the United States following Reconstruction. At this time the racial question was constructed differently there than in Europe. If in the European tradition Jews were equated with Blacks, in the United States they clearly were not Blacks, even though they were understood as different. Twain's early image of the diseased Jew, and its relationship to models of Jewish 'infiltration' into other arenas of modern life, such as the economy, is reversed for his contemporary American readers. In an exchange of letters in 1874, in the prestigious Philadelphia *Medical and Surgical Reporter*, Madison Marsh, a physician from Port Hudson, Lousiana, put forth the argument that Jews had a much greater toleration for disease than the general population. He based his view on the supposed Jewish immunity from tuberculosis. Marsh argued that the Jews 'enjoy a wonderful national immunity from, not only phthisis [tuberculosis] but all disease of the thoracic viscera'.[23] The Jew does not suffer from tuberculosis because 'his constitution has become so hardened and fortified against disease by centuries of national calamities, by the dietetics, regimen and sanitas of his religion, continuing for consecutive years of so many ages'.[24] This view was generally held during the latter half of the nineteenth century. Lucian Wolf, in a debate before the Anthropological Society of Great Britain and Ireland in 1885, stated categorically that 'figures could also be given to prove the immunity of Jews from phthisis', and Dr Asher, in that same debate, observed that 'Jews had an extraordinary power of resistance to phthisis'.[25] Jews (at least Jews in the Diaspora) live longer, have a lower child mortality, and are generally healthier than Christians. The Jew's 'high average physique . . . is not less remarkable than the high average of his intelligence'.[26] Jews are the 'purest, finest, and most perfect type of the Caucasian race'.[27]

This view was widely espoused by American Jews in the late nineteenth century. Rabbi Joseph Krauskopf informed his Reformed congregation in Philadelphia that

Eminent physicians and statisticians have amply confirmed the truth: that the marvelous preservation of Israel, despite all the efforts to blot them out from the face of the earth, their comparative freedom from a number of diseases, which cause frightful ravages among the Non-Jewish people, was largely due to their close adherence to their excellent Sanitary Laws. Health was their coat of mail, it was their magic shield that caught, and warded off, every thrust aimed at their heart. Vitality was their birthright. . . . Their immunity, which the enemy charged to magic-Arts, to alliances with the spirits of evil, was traceable solely to their faithful compliance with the sanitary requirements of their religion.[28]

Marsh added one new twist to this equation: Jews are healthier, live longer, are more immune to disease, are more intelligent because of their healthful practices, such as diet, and the fact that they belong to the 'white' race. Or at least so the Jew was seen by this rural Louisiana physician during Reconstruction.

A month after this report was published, it was answered in detail by Ephraim M. Epstein, a Jewish physician practicing in Cincinnati, Ohio, who had earlier practiced medicine in Vienna and in Russia. He rebutted Marsh's argument point by point: Jews have no immunity from tuberculosis, or any other disease, including those long associated with Jewish religious practices: 'I am sure I have observed no Jewish immunity from any disease, venereal disease not excepted'.[29] Jews do not have 'superior longevity', they have no advantage either because of their diet or because of their practice of circumcision. But Jews do possess a quality lacking in their Christian neighbours. What makes Jews less at risk is the network of support, the 'close fraternity, one Jew never forsaking the material welfare of his brother Jew, and he knows it instinctively'.[30] It is indeed the 'common mental construction' of the Jew which preserves his health. And, in addition, 'the constitutional stamina which that nation inherited from its progenitor, Abraham of old, and because it kept that inheritance undeteriorated by not intermarrying with other races'.[31] Group dynamics and racial purity are the source of Jewish health, such as it is.

Here the battle was joined: the Southern, Christian physician saw in the Jews' social practices and their race a key to universal health. Marsh, of course, defines race in terms of his own ideological understanding of the primary difference between the 'Negro' and the 'Caucasian' races. The Jews, according to the standard textbooks of the period, such as that of the Viennese biologist Carl Claus, are indeed 'Caucasians'.[32] But in American terms, following the close of the Civil War, this concept was given a special, intensely political association. Whites have the potential with good diet and the fortitude to bear oppression (such as Reconstruction), to be healthier, more intelligent, more immune from disease than – and here Marsh's reader's would understand – than . . . Blacks. The Eastern European Jewish physician saw any limited advantage accruing to the Jews lying in their inherited nature and sexual practices to which the non-Jews could have absolutely no access, indeed which by definition exclude them.

Marsh's intensely vituperative response came in August of 1874.[33] Initially, he called on statistical evidence from Prussian, French and British sources to buttress his argument about Jewish longevity. He then dismissed Epstein's argument about Jewish susceptibility to disease completely and turned to the importance of what Epstein had called 'the moral cause that had prevented intermarriage of the Jews with other nations, and thus preserved intact their health and tenacity of life' (p. 133). It was circumcision as a sign of the separateness and selectivity of the Jews that Epstein evoked as the proof for his case about Jewish difference. Circumcision for Marsh is a 'sanitary measure and religious rite . . . in practice by the ancient Egyptians. . . . It never became a Hebrew institution until friendly relations had been established between Abraham and the Egyptians. Then it was initiated by the circumcision of Abraham and Isaac by the express command of God' (p. 133). Circumcision was an Egyptian ritual, and 'Moses, the great champion, leader and lawgiver of the Hebrew race, was himself an Egyptian priest, educated in all the deep research and arts of the Chaldean Mage and mystic philosophic development of Egyptian and Oriental science, and all that was then known of the science of medicine, in its general principles and in its application of details for the preservation of health and prevention of disease' (p. 133). It is this philosophy, with 'a slight tinge of Egyptian and Indian, or Asiatic philosophy, and shadow of its teachings [which] pervade all the books of Moses' (p. 133). The ritual practices of the Jews are but an amalgam of the combined knowledge of the West. They are in no way the special product of this inbred and haughty people. And indeed, Marsh, like Mark Twain, is immediately brought back to Egypt, to the 'damp and cobwebby mold of antiquity', the space where Christian Americans envision Jews.

What could Epstein know about real medicine? Marsh simply dismisses Epstein as merely a Jew, whose authority is solely drawn from this fact: 'What evidence or authority does he bring to support his pretensions to superior knowledge? His being himself a Jew, per se . . .' (p. 134). And he affirmed his view that the Jews possessed the secret to greater health which they were unwilling to share with the rest of the world. The subtext to Marsh's argument is that the Jews' special immunity is the result of historic accident. But the true secret is that this gift is not theirs at all; it was taken from the peoples among whom they lived. Jews such as Epstein are charlatans who try to disguise their true nature. In the nineteenth century it was often the special nature of the Jew's body that lay at the core of anti-Semitism. In the late nineteenth century it was the claim for the special nature of the Jewish body that provoked anger toward the Jews' sexual selectivity or *amixia*.[34] Marsh turns this about, as he, too, wished to share in the special status of the 'healthy' Jewish body.

Circumcision had become a major issue for American medicine. Indeed, the American physician Peter Charles Remondino, writing in the 1870s, could note that 'circumcision is like a substantial and well-secured life annuity . . . it ensures them better health, greater capacity for labour, longer life, less nervousness, sickness, loss of time . . .'.[35] And indeed, by the 1890s, an American association had begun to be made between 'uncircumcised' and 'uncivilised'.[36] In this context it is of little surprise that circumcision, an intervention which could be made by the physician, came to have a function in the definition of 'hygiene'. But it is in no way to be understood as a Jewish practice, in the terms which Epstein had outlined. The debates about the 'health' or 'illness' of the Jews centred on the inherent nature or social practices of the Jews. The image of the Jew as different was always stated in the context of an unstated understanding that the African-American had a diseased and inferior nature. Twain's views about the diseased nature of the Jews in Biblical times can be placed within this long-standing and complex debate about where the true boundary of inferiority is to be placed. Twain's focus on the religious aspects of disease and the corrupt body reflects the parameters of this debate. Like Marsh, Twain sees the world through the Christian model of the nature of the Jew. The Jew is different from the Christian in terms of the very nature of his body.

Twain sees the Diseased Jew

The contrast between the Jews Mark Twain represents in his essay of 1898 and those he saw in 1867 is striking. In the *Adventures of Huckleberry Finn* he had parodied white American assumptions about the relationship between African-Americans and mental illness, assumptions that dominated the medical discourse about African-Americans from the 1840s on through Reconstruction.[37] In his 1898 essay on the Jews, written during anti-Semitic outbreaks in the United States and in the light of the debates he had experienced in Vienna, he seems to take a more liberal, benign view of the Jews. Indeed, the late 1890s marks the high point of both anti-Semitic and anti-African-American hysteria.[38] Certainly they, like Nigger Jim, are in no way to be associated with images of disease. Or at least not overtly. For Twain's concern in the 1890s is to present a positive image of the Jew's sense of communal responsibility. For Twain, the Jews may still be diseased, like other peoples, but they at least take care of their own. The Jews are never beggars; indeed, they create 'charitable institutions' like hospitals (p. 14) to take care of their afflicted. They are quite unlike the diseased multitudes that had flocked to the tent of the Western doctor in Palestine some three decades earlier.

For these Jews are the victims of society. As Susy Clemens recorded in her notebook: 'he [Twain] decided that the Jews had always seemed to him a race much to be respected; also they had suffered much, and had been greatly persecuted, so to ridicule or make fun of them seemed to be like attacking a man who was already down'.[39] The debate between those who believed that illness was an essential aspect of the Jewish race and those who saw it as a reflection of the social status of the Jews is worked out in Twain's own texts. Twain saw, at the *fin de siècle*, the Jews as formed by neither space nor race, but by their oppression by Western culture.

The rationale for his essay on the Jews in 1898 was a letter from a

Jewish-American lawyer asking Twain about the cause of anti-Semitism. The Jews are seen by Twain as the victims, especially in the context of his experience in Vienna. Twain sees contemporary Jews as little different from all of the other inhabitants of Europe and the United States, except that they are aware of their victimization. Once Twain moved from the past to the present some 30 years later, the argument shifted from one about the origins of Christianity to the nature of late nineteenth-century capitalism and the role of the Jews. But these two aspects of the Jew as the point of origin of Christianity and capitalism are linked, as we have seen in the arguments about the Jew's nature in the eighteenth and nineteenth centuries. Initially the Jews were, for Twain, the afflicted and superstitious Jews of the past: Naaman the Leper, incarnate in Twain's experience entering the Holy Land. These Jews are thus the originators of Christianity. But the miracles of Christ, recounted in detail in Twain's commentary, seem not to have helped them very much over time. For they seem still to be in the same diseased state as they were 2000 years before Twain arrived in the Holy Land. It appeared, then, to be American science that the sufferers in the Holy Land needed, rather than the mysteries of the past.

Twain differentiated between the corrupt Jews of the Bible and contemporary Jewry. But also, unconsciously, he linked them. Twain found it impossible to hold these two categories apart. In his essay of 1898 Twain invokes his experience with Jews in the South and noted that 'religion [i.e. Christianity] had nothing to do with the hatred of the Jew'. During Reconstruction, the Jew had opened 'shop on the plantation, supplied all the Negro's wants on credit, and at the end of the season was proprietor of the Negro's share of the present crop and of part of the share of the next one. Before long, the whites detested the Jew, and it is doubtful if the Negro loved him' (p. 18). The category 'Jew' is not religious, as Marsh noted, but racial. In his system Twain, like Marsh, can differentiate between 'whites', 'Negroes' and 'Jews'. Jews are designated as different from 'whites' and 'Negroes' on the basis of their racially marked character and practices. Here the question is whether the Jew was white or not, a question that reappeared in the debate about the social position of the Jew in the South during the Leo Frank case.[40] This distinction is important. For just as Twain needed to separate his identity from that of the diseased Jews and their progeny in the Middle East, so too does he need to see himself as different from American Jews. For as Clara Clemens commented, Twain's 'eloquent . . . defense of Christ's race' was turned so that 'it was rumored at one time Father himself was a Jew'.[41]

Indeed in Vienna, while he was observing the debates which triggered the essay on the Jews, he was labelled by the anti-Semitic press as the 'Jew Mark Twain'.[42] Just as Twain needed to create a diseased inheritance for the Jews in the 1860s, so too does he need to distinguish himself from the corrupt Jews of the 1890s.

The Jews are diseased, but their infection is the desire for capital. Twain's answer to anti-Semitism returns to the central theme of his earlier writing, to the image of the Jews in the Holy Land. Twain supports the political aims of Theodor Herzl. But ironically he fears the ingathering 'in Palestine, with a government of their own – under the suzerainty of the Sultan, I suppose'. For 'if that concentration of the cunningest brains in the world was going to be made in a free country (bar Scotland), I think it would be politic to stop it. It will not be well to let that race find out its strength. If the horses knew theirs, we should not ride any more' (p. 27). It is this cunning that marked the Jews in the South and it is this cunning which Twain sensed in the origins of Christianity. And this cunning is a sign of the inherent difference of the Jews as a race, a mark of their corruption and disease. For in the science of the late nineteenth century, this corrupt genius is as certain a pathological sign as are the physical symptoms of the leper.[43] Twain's rhetoric about physical disease has been transformed into the rhetoric about psychological predisposition, which is as far as he was able to go in rethinking the meaning of the diseases of the Jews. Twain sees the diseases of the Jews as markers for the Jews' difference, but also for the difference which they (as individuals who have experienced death and disease in their own world) see in themselves. And yet, in his own estimation, he is not as 'ill' as the Jews and that redeems him.

6 The Beautiful Body and AIDS: The Image of the Body at Risk at the Close of the Twentieth Century

Beautiful and Healthy Bodies?

At the close of the twentieth century the opposition of the healthy and erotic to the diseased and ugly has developed in new and often surprising ways in the context of AIDS. Indeed, Simon Whatney, in 1987, looked at AIDS as presenting 'a crisis of representation itself, a crisis over the entire framing of knowledge about the human body and its capacities for sexual pleasure'.[1] Having sketched some of the presuppositions that existed at the turn of the century and beyond about the meaning of the ugly body as a sign of disease, not only of the body but of the psyche or character, and the struggle by groups, such as Jews, to overcome their sense of the insufficiency of their bodies through medical intervention, we can turn to a new vocabulary of images consciously associated with a 'new' disease, AIDS, which wrestled with the discourse of the ugly, unerotic body and soul from the very identification of the disease.[2]

In my earlier work on AIDS I compared the incomparable – the meaning of different diseases in different historical epochs and national contexts – with only one (I believe) major similarity, that they are both understood only as incurable, sexually transmitted illnesses.[3] Simon Whatney spoke of the new 'equation of sex with AIDS which stands to construct a new contagion theory of homosexuality' (p. 132). But the subsequent historiography of the visual representation of AIDS has drawn on even more than the history of homosexuality in the West for its models. Here I want to add the question of the continuity and transformation of the meaning of the beautiful to the general as well as medical contexts of the illness. I will examine visual representations of illness in the arena of public health information across a number of cultural realms (and national contexts) to see whether the visual representation of the person at risk from or with AIDS can be understood as an aestheticized one. All of these aestheticized images attempt to simplify the lived complexity of disease through the use of highly constructed visual images.

We shall be examining the vocabulary of the images in the public health posters collected over the past five years in the National Library of Medicine at Bethesda, Maryland, which contains the largest collection of poster art dealing with questions of health in the United States.[4] As part of this collection of 3500 images, 1100 posters dealing specifically with AIDS and HIV infection have been amassed by William Helfand, who is consultant to the collection.[5] This collection exhaustively covers the decade of the 1980s and is presently ongoing, bringing the AIDS posters of the 1990s together in a single place. I examined and categorized 700 posters. The images reproduced here represent the tendencies found in the analysis of all the images examined, whether or not discussed. Not all of these posters represent the body, even as an abstraction, but I focus on those that do.

Using this collection, I have been able to document the public image of the body in advertising dealing with AIDS from its popular discovery in the early 1980s to today. The images are all posters, that is, they were all intended for public display, and were all intended to communicate specific information directly to a mass audience. The posters presume a certain level of awareness of AIDS; therefore reading the posters provides an index of awareness of the disease, the images used to evoke the disease, the visual and verbal language employed to characterize those who have or are at risk from the disease, and an index of how the disease was understood over time and in various visual cultures both within and outside of the United States. While many of the posters are American, there are enough sources from beyond the United States to have enabled me to undertake a truly comparative study. The organizations that generated this material widely diverge in their funding sources or institutional structure, ranging from official state agencies responsible for the public's health to private, single-issue foundations.

Thus the posters are not 'anonymous' folk art, but the products of a sophisticated advertising culture (whether they were or not designed and circulated by official 'advertising' agencies) that has specific assumptions about its audience and that audience's capacity for the quick assimilation of information as well as the best means to communicate this information. This culture of public health advertising, as we shall see, builds on notions of health and beauty, ugliness and disease, in complicated ways. We assume that these posters have an overt 'intention'. We can explore what this intention was and how the visual and verbal vocabulary selected was appropriate, for that overt intention masked covert assumptions that may or may not vitiate the original intention. These images have presumed audiences, visual vocabularies and intended contexts other than the high art representations of AIDS during this same period.[6] The 1988 AIDS art exhibit in Berlin already presented a wide range of international work, such as Peter Hujar's photographs of himself dying of AIDS or Mark Golebiowski's photographs of AIDS activists in wheelchairs protesting at the American Food and Drug Administration.[7] Such images rarely overlapped with the public health images, in which death is present as an abstraction, if at all, and never as a daily reality. Missing in the posters is the postmodern, but really the post-Shoah notion of death, 'already represented in objects, persons, time, and desire'.[8] They reject mourning as an oppropriate mode of dealing with the anxiety about the self. It is the repression of mourning that kills the anxiety about the death of the self represented by the memory of the death of the Other. Missing also is the anger and the anxiety of writers such as the gay German novelist Mario Wirz, born 1956, who laments the internalization of the notion of the diseased, dangerous, and therefore ugly, body of the person with AIDS:

I am not yet stupid enough to regret the years of pleasure. I feel the hunger of these nights with all of the memory of all of the warm bodies, which I fled to. Ashes over my foolish attempts to justify myself, all the bad grades which were given men. The virus wolf is howling in the night. I am afraid of death and I am afraid of dying. Paranoia in the cobwebs on the ceiling. My head, a single horror video. I awake in my coffin. I cry and fight my way through the unforgiving wood and the earth.[9]

Here the anxiety about illness marks the soul. The specific notion of the body of the person with AIDS as marked in such a way as to make it visible is found in a number of first-hand accounts of the illness. In a passage later deleted from his autobiography, George Whitmore described his response to his own body:

My body. I hadn't looked at it much.
Before I left for New Hampshire, at the Passover seder with my lover Michael's family, we took turns reading the Haggadah in booklets illustrated with line drawings. When we reached the page with the plagues God brought down on the Egyptians, there was a locust, there was a dead fish with x's for eyes, there was the outline of a man with dots all over him, signifying boils. I stared at the cartoon of the man with the boils. I knew Michael, sitting next to me, was thinking the same thing. My body was like that now. I'd had three lesions 12 months before. Now there were three dozen.
One day in New Hampshire, in the shower, I looked at my body. It was as if I'd never seen it before.
A transformation had taken place and it was written on my skin.[10]

This is missing or mediated in the world of the public health image.[11] Irony is also missing from that source. The 'SPEW Homographic

Convergence' shows in Chicago (1992) and Los Angeles (1993), for example, employ a very different set of images to represent the world, often parodies of gay pornography, than do the rather selfconsciously unironic images of the public health world – no matter what their ideological provenance.[12]

Central to my analysis of these public health posters is a close reading of their iconography, their visual vocabulary. Here the image – as in the nineteenth century – provides its own referents that delineate and make specific certain arguments by what is omitted as well as by what is included. The tracing of specific visual themes, the question of who and what is represented (and not represented) on the posters and how they are portrayed gives us a vocabulary of images that is tied closely to the image of AIDS and HIV infection. The representation of the person at risk of infection, infected with the HIV virus or the person with AIDS that results, can provide us with a clear understanding of how these categories are ideologically presented.

We can also question whether specific tendencies in the public image of AIDS realized their intention to inform the target group(s) or led to the desired behaviour(s). Some scholarly work has been undertaken to evaluate specific projects, such as the special 1989 issue on AIDS and communication of the *AIDS and Public Policy Journal* as well as the special 1989 number of *October* on AIDS. However, only the catalogue by Douglas Crimp offers any comparable critical overview of this material.[13] At present there are few studies that have either the extensive database of this one or that provide this type of detailed analysis.[14] But rather than ask whether exposure to a specific image actually altered any single individual's or presumed collective's behaviour, I shall address the complex and often contradictory vocabulary of images present in the posters themselves. It is clearly impossible to isolate the effect of the exposure to a single image. Rather, a critical analysis of the cultural presuppositions present in the poster will allow us to gauge the complex and often contradictory messages being presented to various overlapping thought collectives.

What immediately strikes a viewer coming to the 'mass' world of the public health poster from the 'high art' world of 'AIDS art' is the virtual absence of images of the diseased body. The posters represent, when they represent human beings at all, three categories. There are numerous images of people at risk as well as people who are HIV-positive, and some very few representations of death as an abstraction. Our earlier discussion of the cultural expectation that the ill body will be visually marked as ugly makes it striking that these posters represent the body at risk and even the ill body as beautiful, even erotic. Death certainly threatens, but dying itself is absent. While death is present, dying is absent. What are striking is how the image of the body at risk and the ill body in the world of the public health posters parallel one another, and the limited context in which even the symbolic representation of the mask of death is evoked. Only rarely is the question of a visually compromised body evoked.

The rationale for this avoidance seems clear. The classic model of 'health/beauty' and 'illness/ugliness' is part of the cultural baggage that accompanies any representation of the ill or healthy body. Associated with that model is its moral dimension. Then the historical context of the meaning of AIDS and its powerful association with homosexual activity must be added as a second subtext for these images. The healthy in this model cannot be the homosexual, who has been medicalized as pathological since at least the middle of the nineteenth century. Indeed, the movement to depathologize homosexuality that began in the 1960s needed to create quite the opposite image. The homosexual is not only not 'ill' but 'healthy', is not 'ugly' but 'beautiful'. The image of the homosexual, especially in the light of the association of AIDS and homosexuality, becomes eroticized to counter the conventional association of homosexuality with deviancy and disease. The collective in this case is no longer the 'general culture' (self-defined), but the world of the homosexual that must be preserved and seen as healthy. This is quite the antithesis of the older, popular image of homosexuality in the general culture as transmitted by the Western media.

The anxiety about illness as a danger to the collective is repressed in a continuation of the older model of 'health/beauty' and 'illness/ugliness'. The person at risk but uninfected by HIV is 'healthy' and therefore beautiful, and poses no danger to the collective's continuity. The person with an HIV infection, however, is the focus of anxiety about individual as well as collective death and decay. This person is a reminder of the necessary presence of death even in a seemingly healthy world. Such an image becomes the locus of 'sympathy' and 'identification' as a means of combating the anxiety that this category evokes. Everyone will die, the argument goes, and the only way we can deal with death is by constructing categories that deny dying – such as 'beauty/health'. Thus the persons with AIDS (PWAS) in these images are both dying and not really dying. The anxiety about death can be thus bounded.

A corollary seems to be true of this corpus of images – even the infected body, the body that overtly signifies its potential for death and therefore provokes our anxiety about dying, must be so constructed that it denies the potential of dying. For if the body at risk is the healthy body (by definition), the infected body should be the ill body and should be ugly and diseased, if not in its present state then in its future state, to show that it is not beautiful and healthy. This would continue the older, general model of deviancy and disease associated with the homoerotic and by extension with other 'groups' defined as risk groups. One way of countering this is to create the argument that everyone is part of an at-risk group. Each body that constitutes this 'everyone' must be 'beautiful/healthy'. The answer is to see the potentially ill body only in terms of the iconography of the healthy body at risk. Here it is not to highlight the potential for illness but to link this category with that of the healthy body, the body that does not provide any risk for the collective. This denies the older association of the homoerotic body that was seemingly 'beautiful/healthy' on the surface yet was understood to contain within it the seeds of its own corruption and death.

The ill body with its visual clues that point to the disease process (defined as ugly) is missing from this iconography. But the dead body is present. The dead body is the antithesis of 'health/beauty'; it is 'illness/ugliness'. It is not only non-erotic but presents an anti-body, a body completely separate from the erotic, living body. The reduction of the body to the skeleton is the reduction to the overtly symbolic. Here the medieval tradition of the *memento mori* or the early modern one of *Et in arcadia ego* – 'Even in Arcadia, there am I' (spoken by Death) – is evoked to separate the 'erotic/beautiful/healthy' body with its commitment to the continuity of the group from the terminated/grotesque/ dead one.[15] This is not the eroticized corpse that one finds in male fantasies about the female body.[16] The erotic body, no matter what its actual status, remains associated with the healthy, not with the dead or dying. Dying is excluded, as it forms a transition between the 'infected' category and the iconography of death. Death, represented by the icon of the skeletal body, is separated from all the categories of life and of the perpetuation of the group. For here the evocation of death using the iconography of the dead/ugly is clear. The vocabulary of images found in this material is shaped by the older view of the antithesis of 'health/beauty' and 'illness/ugliness'. And yet it restructures it so as to make it applicable to new social images and cultural belief systems.

The Body at Risk

The body at risk is clearly the eroticized body. It is a youthful body. It is the beautiful body of the advertising agency interested in selling a new product – safe sex. But the function of the eroticization of the body, especially the male body, seems always to be tinged with a sense of anxiety or guilt. Certainly the *locus classicus* for this in the world of the public health poster is the widely circulated United States Public Health Service image of the young man and a sock. This rather self-embarrassed poster presents a photograph, placed slightly off-centre, of a fully clothed, slightly built seated male putting on a sock with the motto 'Putting on a condom is just as simple' (illus. 53). Here a series of associations are made in a highly censored and rather fetishistic vocabulary – the foot replaces the penis, the sock the condom, the clothed body the naked (but not nude) body. The very angle of the photograph throws our gaze on the image of a second chair on which rests the (a) second sock. The reference is opaque, even if the intent is clear. The second sock represents a second condom, i.e., the offstage presence of a male partner. This poster (and the parallel television advertisement) came quickly to be the brunt of jokes on national television reflecting of the innate prudery of the representation.[17]

An answer to this type of symbolic representation of the individual at risk in the images of safe sex has been to 'eroticize the condom', rather than to symbolize it. A photographic image from the San Francisco AIDS Foundation from 1988 represents a nude (not naked) male with an erect penis sheathed in a condom (illus. 54). The body alone is presented, the head is masked by the frame (except for the mouth) so as to emphasis the muscular, healthy, erotic male body. This is a very different body from that of the sock advertisement. It sits at the centre of the image, and is muscular and dominant rather than bowed and subservient. The eroticized male body is directed at a male gaze, as it uses the conventions of the soft-porn or erotic photographs of the male body from Western gay culture.[18] Therefore no partner is represented, as the viewer is the implied partner.

A sexualized, nude body does not need a head as long as it has a mouth, as the erotic pose emphasizes the relationship between mouth and penis. The anonymity of the eroticized male body in a beefcake pose evokes sexuality but also danger. A British poster presents a photograph of an exposed male torso which is labelled 'AIDS is in town – *don't* pass it on' (illus. 55). Here, too, the eroticized position of the subject, torso exposed, undershirt pulled up over the pectorals, thumbs hooked in the pockets of tight jeans, evokes the male viewer. But the phrase 'AIDS is in town' literally replaces the head of the image. If the San Francisco poster places its message between the legs of the male to deliver its message about safe sex, then the British poster uses it as a cartoon balloon, presenting the presumed thoughts of the sexualized torso. Indeed, even in the African-American community the evocation of this masculinity at risk uses the beefcake approach, although desiring to evoke older images of enslavement and powerlessness (illus. 56). A poster by the South Carolina Coalition of Black Church Leaders used the drawing of a muscular slave in chains (in a tobacco field), upper torso bare, dressed in torn-off pants, to stress that one should not be 'Bound by the chains of ignorance – learn about AIDS'. It is as if the evocation of the slave, so permanent a part of the African-American historical vocabulary, represented a return to an older well-known image of risk associated with the African-American male.

All of these images, no matter how varied they are in their context, represent healthy if not beautiful bodies. Condom education is likewise tied to the image of the healthy male body in a state of partial undress. One poster from the Health Education Resource Organization in Maryland represents two males, one partially removing his undershirt in a photograph with the motto 'You won't believe what we like to wear in bed' (illus. 57). Likewise, the Canadian 'Play safe this summer' poster features a drawing of two beefcake males caressing while stripped to the waist before a giant safety pin (illus. 58). The informal 'pickup' in a train in a Swedish poster presents a photograph of two clothed men with the warning 'You get all of his experiences' (illus. 59). Being clothed (i.e. wearing a condom) evokes the notion of being safe from danger. A parallel Norwegian image of two smiling nude males, placed front to back, with the motto 'Joy is caring' cuts them off well above the waist (illus. 60). The image of the partially clothed male, whether clothed in jeans or in a condom or without socks, comes to represent safe sex, sex with condoms.[19] The eroticization of the body is intended to carry over into the eroticization of the act of safe sex. Again the viewer is 'told' that being partially clothed is better than being unclothed, which is, of course, the not so subtle message of beefcake images anyway. That which is hidden is that which is eroticized. Such messages can be presented in various guises.[20]

It is clearly not only the homoerotic that is sensualized in AIDS public health posters; heterosexual posters employ the same tropes of clothing and eroticization of the body. In a poster from the Danish National Board of Health, a photograph of a scene of heterosexual sexuality, elegantly backlit, with the motto 'Sex is beautiful' (illus. 61), the female is nude, but the male is clothed in jeans. Here the male's body as the protected/ing partner is made equivalent to his penis. In the heterosexual images in a French poster, the male is actually reduced to a condom. 'He' as a disembodied voice (represented by a rolled condom) complains to 'her' about wearing a condom and 'she', a photo of a beautiful woman, responds by laughing at his complaint (illus. 62). The

Putting On A Condom Is Just As Simple.

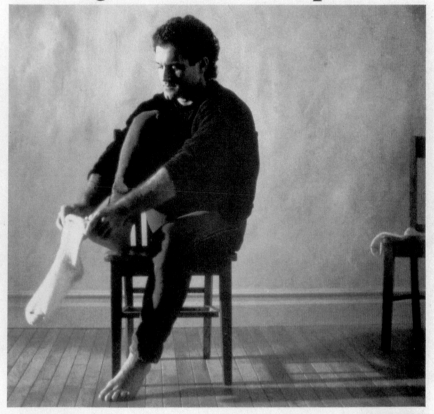

Condoms are one of the simplest and best forms of protection against AIDS. But they're only effective if they are used properly every time you have sex. Why risk not using them? For more information about condoms, AIDS and AIDS prevention, call 1-800-342-AIDS.

53 The United States Public Health Service poster that replaced condom use with footwear.

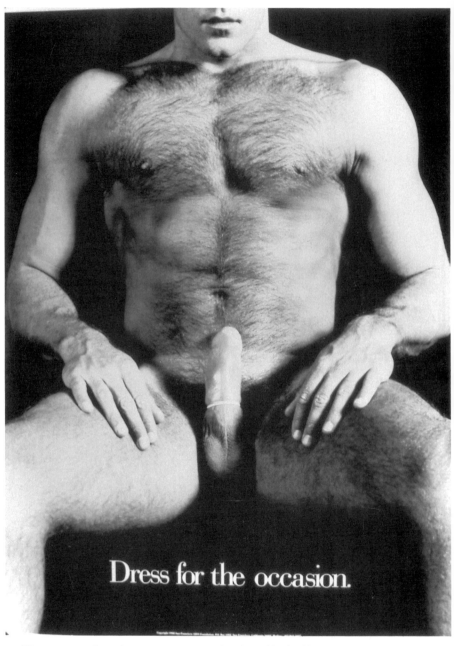

Dress for the occasion.

54 The answer to the embarrassment expressed in the public health poster is answered by the beefcake image in this poster from the San Francisco AIDS Foundation from 1988.

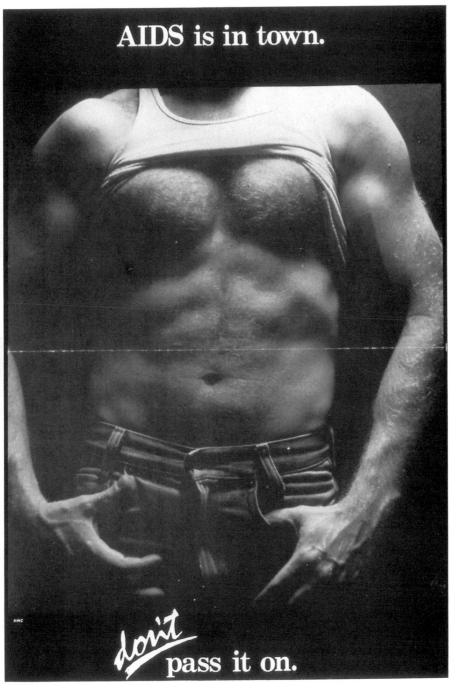

55 A British poster presents a photograph of an exposed male torso that stresses the erotic image of the person at risk.

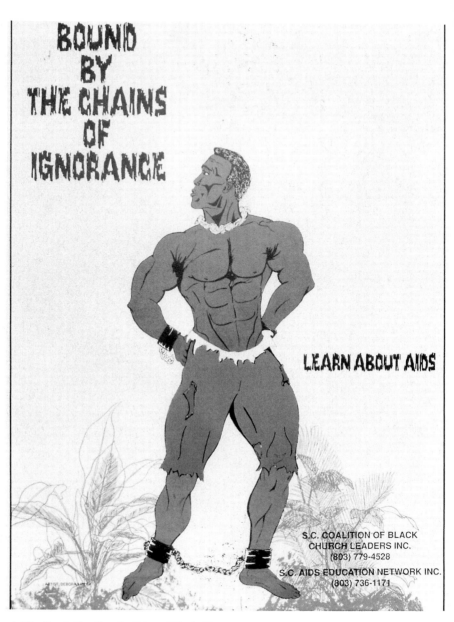

56 The South Carolina Coalition of Black Church Leaders issued this poster in the late 1980s that evoked both the beautiful male body and the image of the African-American in chains.

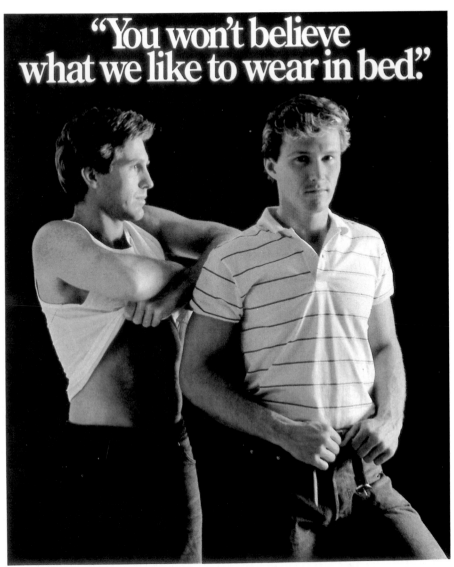

"You won't believe
what we like to wear in bed."

More and more smart men are slipping into condoms
tonight. Protecting themselves and their partners.
And, enjoying sex all over again. Shouldn't you?

Use condoms.
There's living proof they stop AIDS.

945-AIDS • 251-1164 • 1-800-638-6252
Baltimore Metro   DC Metro   Elsewhere in MD
* Design created by Jeff McElhaney. Writer: David Foote. Print Production: Allan Sprecher. Photography for HERO.

57 The Health Education Resource Organization, Maryland, presents a modified
version of the beefcake image of the person at risk in this 1986 poster.

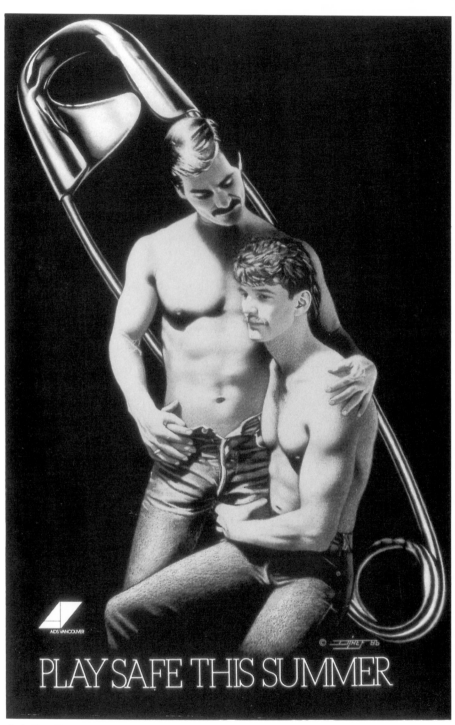

PLAY SAFE THIS SUMMER

58 A Canadian poster of 1986 produced by AIDS Vancouver reading 'Play Safe this Summer', featuring a drawing of two males caressing in the beefcake position.

DU FÅR ALLA HANS ERFARENHETER

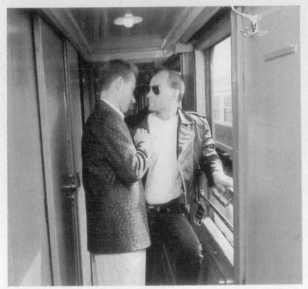

Du kanske bara haft enstaka samlag med andra män. Den du legat med kan däremot ha haft många partners före dig.

Tror du att det finns en risk att du har smittats med HIV, ska du gå och testa dig. Du kan göra det anonymt och behöver inte avslöja något om ditt liv.

Troligen visar testet att du inte är smittad. Då kan du sluta oroa dig både för dig själv och för dina närmaste. Du kan börja ett nytt liv, där du undviker att ta onödiga risker.

RING AIDS-JOUREN 020-78 44 40 OM DU VILL FRÅGA

Du kan fråga om HIV-test och allt annat som rör HIV och AIDS, och få svar och råd av en professionellt utbildad människa från frivilliga stödorganisationen Noaks Ark. Du behöver inte säga vem du är eller lämna några andra upplysningar. 020-numret innebär att du kan ringa överallt ifrån i Sverige och prata så länge du vill, till kostnaden för bara en samtalsmarkering.

59 A Swedish poster with a photograph of two clothed men and the warning 'You get all of his experiences'.

Glede og omsorg

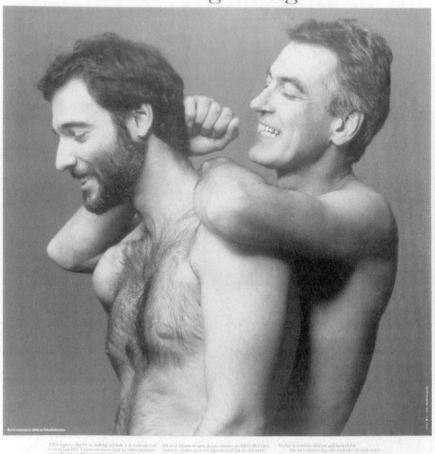

60 A Norwegian poster with a photograph of two smiling, nude males front to back with the motto 'Joy is caring'.

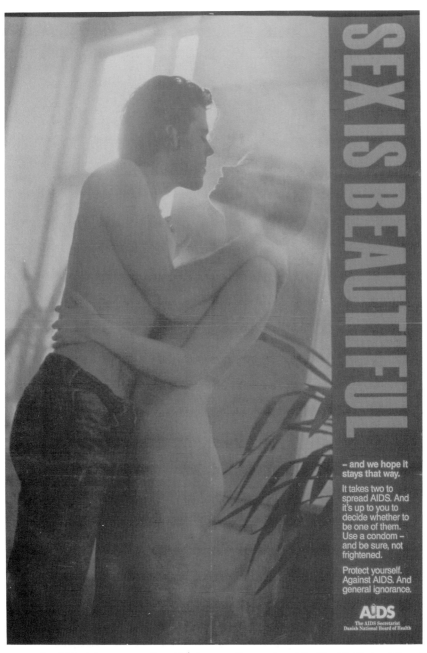

61 A Danish poster produced by the AIDS Secretariat of the Danish National Board of Health with a photograph of a scene of heterosexual sexuality and an English-language text: 'Sex is beautiful'.

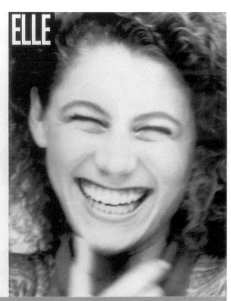

"Il paraît
que
c'est galère
à
mettre"

comité français d'éducation pour la santé

AUJOURD'HUI, LES PRÉSERVATIFS PRÉSERVENT DE TOUT, MÊME DU RIDICULE

62 In this French Public Health Education Committee poster, the male is actually reduced to a condom. 'He', a disembodied voice, complains to 'her' about wearing a condom: It's just so boring using them'; and 'she', a photograph of a beautiful woman, responds by laughing at his complaint.

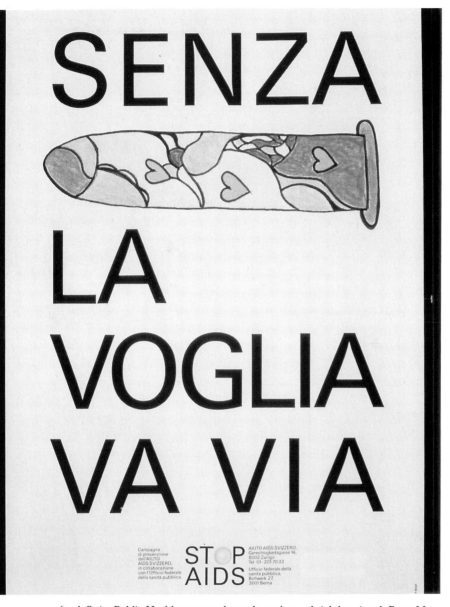

SENZA
LA
VOGLIA
VA VIA

Campagna
di prevenzione
dell'AIUTO
AIDS SVIZZERO,
in collaborazione
con l'Ufficio federale
della sanità pubblica.

ST⚫P
AIDS

AIUTO AIDS SVIZZERO,
Gerechtigkeitsgasse 14,
8002 Zurigo
Tel. 01- 201 70 33
Ufficio federale della
sanità pubblica,
Bollwerk 27,
3001 Berna

63 A Swiss Public Health poster reduces the male to a brightly painted, Peter Max-style condom.

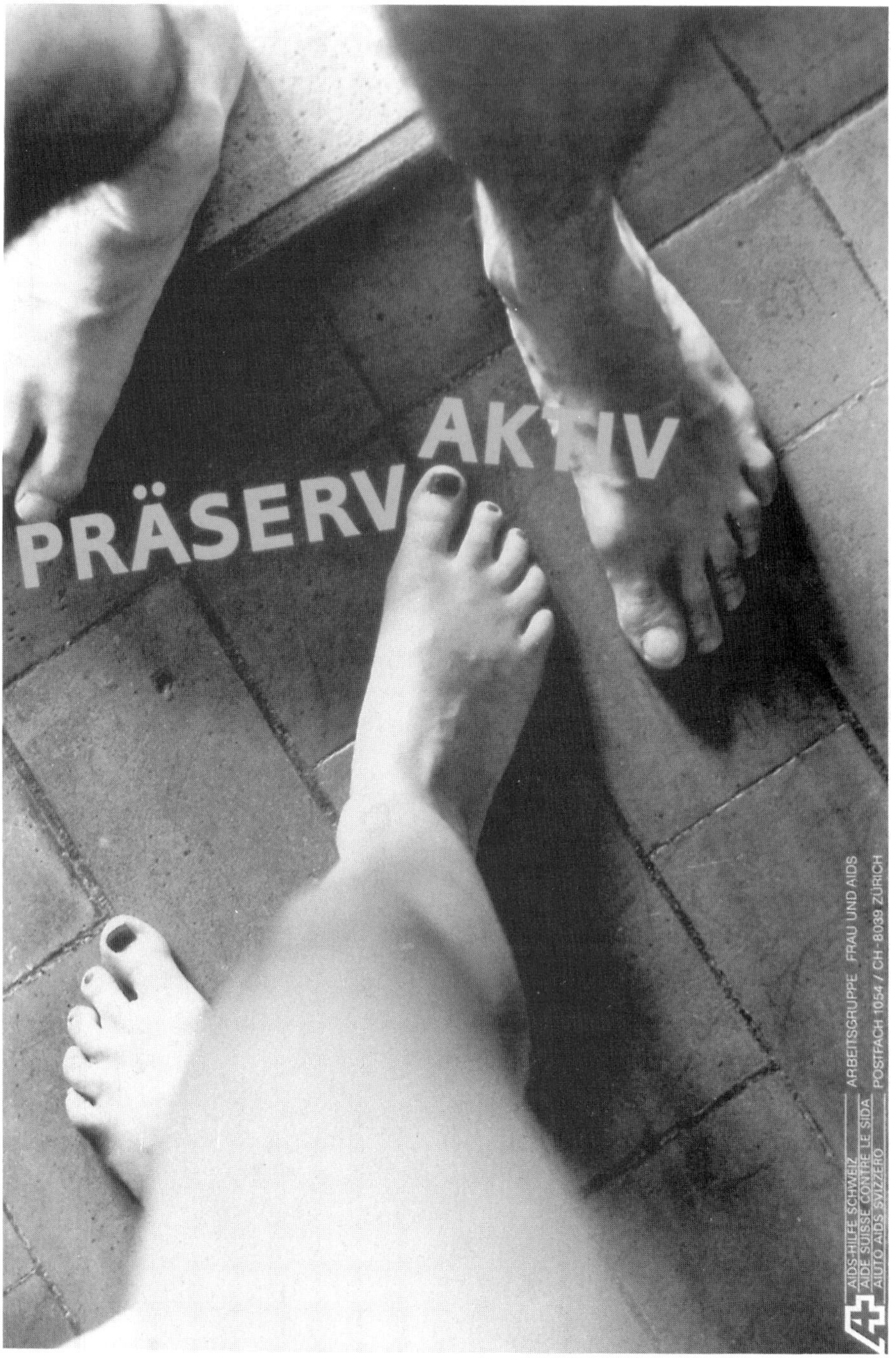
PRÄSERV
AKTIV
AIDS-HILFE SCHWEIZ
AIDE SUISSE CONTRE LE SIDA
AIUTO AIDS SVIZZERO
ARBEITSGRUPPE FRAU UND AIDS
POSTFACH 1054 / CH-8039 ZÜRICH

64 'Prophyl-active': a Swiss AIDS-*Hilfe* poster presents the naked feet of a male and female showing much the same anxiety about the body as the US Public Health 'socks' poster (see illus. 53).

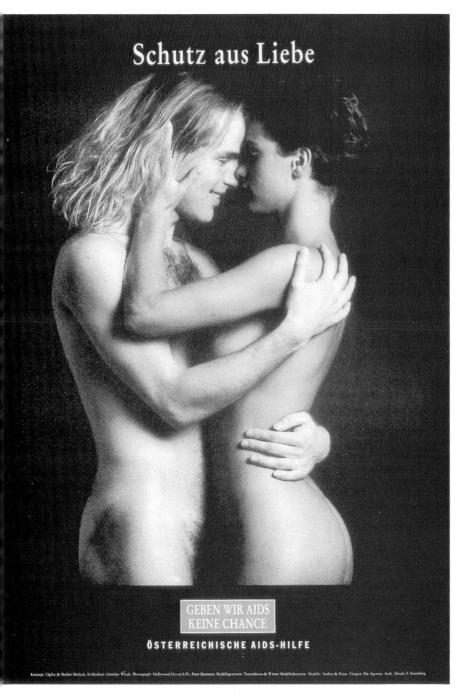

65 'Protect out of love': an Austrian AIDS organization's poster stressing the erotic heterosexual body.

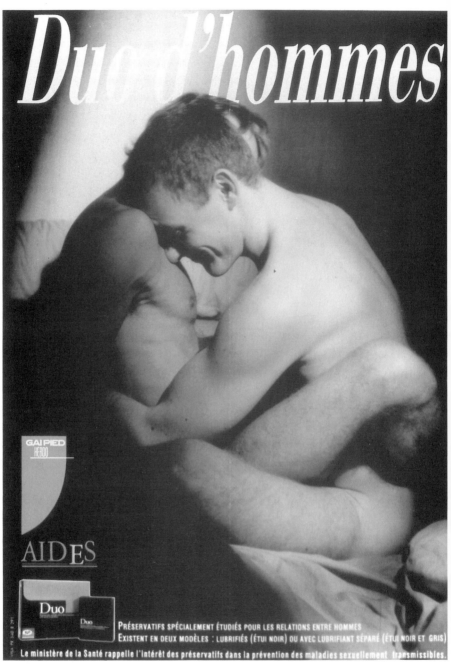

66 French condom advertising picks up the beefcake aspects of the public health posters with their warning label.

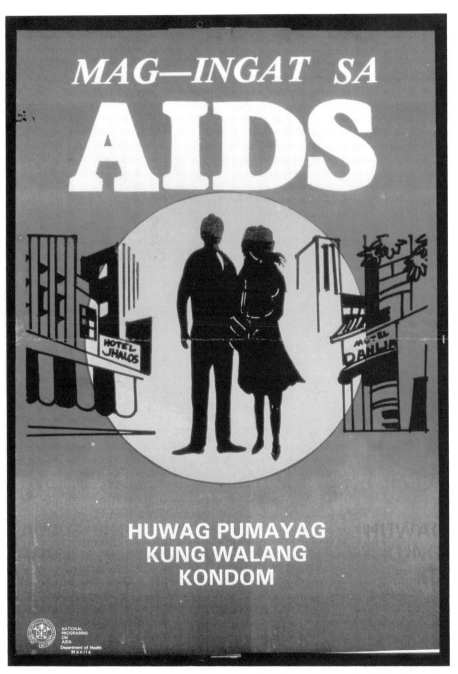

67 'Beware of AIDS – Don't agree to sex if you have no protection': The National Programme on AIDS of the Manila (Philippines) Department of Health places emphasis on heterosexual transmission.

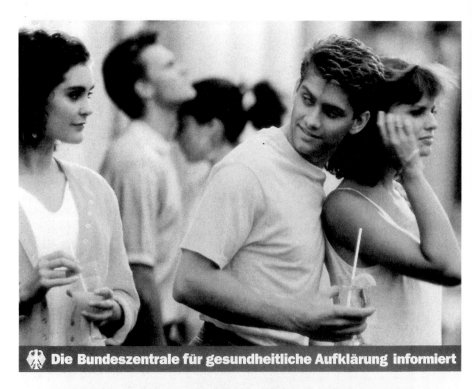

Urlaub von der Treue ist das Ende der Sicherheit.

Aids bekommt man nicht wie einen Schnupfen.

Anstecken kann man sich bei ungeschütztem Sex mit unbekannten Partnern.

Deshalb gilt im Urlaub, wie überall:

Partnerschaftliche Treue ist der beste Schutz vor Aids.

Wenn Sie noch Fragen haben, rufen Sie an: 02 21/89 20 31

GIB AIDS KEINE CHANCE

68 'Holidays from fidelity are the end of safety': The German AIDS-*Hilfe* warns about infidelity.

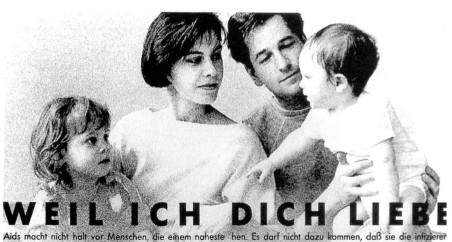

WEIL ICH DICH LIEBE

Aids macht nicht halt vor Menschen, die einem naheste die sie am meisten lieben. Fragen Sie sich, ob Sie ein Risi längst vergessen – heute alles gefährdet, was Ihnen wichtig beraten und testen. Handeln Sie verantwortlich – das sind

hen. Es darf nicht dazu kommen, daß sie die infizierer ko eingegangen sind. Eines, das – vielleicht ist. Wenn Sie nicht sicher sind, lassen Sie sich Sie Ihrem Partner schuldig. Bitte rufen Sie an.

GIB AIDS KEINE CHANCE

Aids-Telefon, Bundeszentrale   für gesundheitliche Aufklärung
☎ 02 21 /   89 20 31
Die Bundesgesund   heitsministerin

69 'Because I love you': The German AIDS-*Hilfe* and the perfect family at risk.

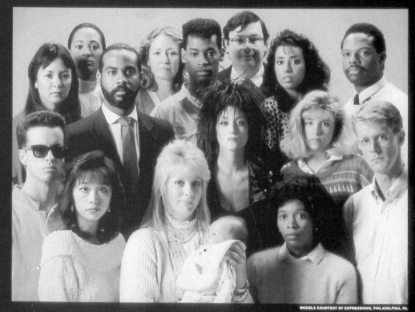

Anyone can get AIDS.

Protect Yourself Use a Condom

If you need help or more information on AIDS call 985-AIDS.
Spread the truth about AIDS.

Philadelphia Department of Public Health
For City of Philadelphia Information and Referral, call 875-6560.

70 In the USA it is not the 'perfect family' but rather the perfect society, balanced carefully to assure the image of a healthy, young, multicultural society. Hidden to the rear of the image is a lank individual with glasses, his hair receding. Ageing and illness lurk even here in the most oblique manner.

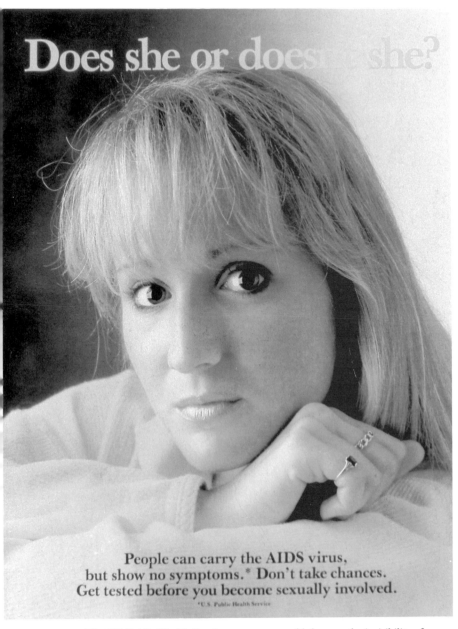

Does she or doesn't she?

People can carry the AIDS virus,
but show no symptoms.* Don't take chances.
Get tested before you become sexually involved.

*U.S. Public Health Service

71 The US Public Health Service returns to an old theme – the invisibility of
illness beneath the beautiful female exterior.

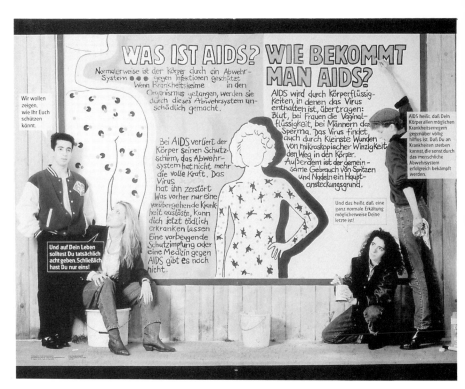

72 A German Ministry of Health, Youth and Women poster of 1989 stressing the education of the teenager concerning the transmission of HIV infection through seemingly perfect skin.

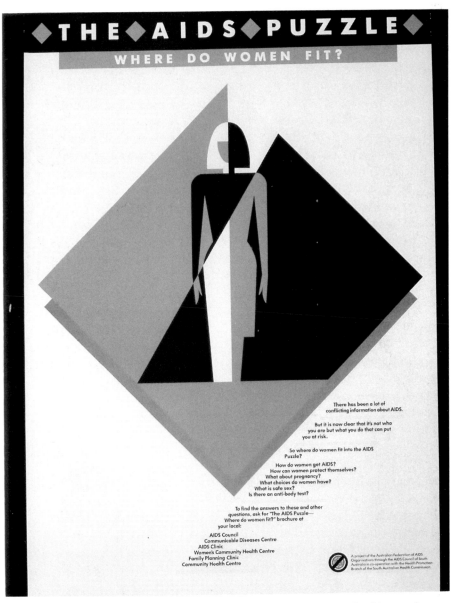

73 The Australian Federation of AIDS Organizations uses a stylized image of a female body to move the image of the person at risk away from the stigmatised male body.

motto is that today a condom prevents everything, even ridicule. The 'Elle' and the 'Lui' evoke the images of the chic up-market magazines of those names, and the labels are placed in such a way as to present the images as magazine covers. An Italian-Swiss public health poster reduces the male to a brightly painted Peter Max-style condom shielding a missing, but clearly erect penis (illus. 63). The male in these images is reduced to his parts, but these parts remain invisible. Yet even this 'invisible' body, its very imagined presence, is healthy and joyful – an ongoing theme in representing the body at risk. Sexuality is enjoyment – but, says the subtext – it is also risk-taking. The infected body, the ill but unmarked body, is displaced onto the image of the condom as a sign of illness. A poster from the Swiss AIDS-*Hilfe* presents the naked feet of a male and a female shot from above with the label 'Prophyl-active' (illus. 64).[21] This effects the same displacement as the socks in the poster we discussed earlier. Here the uncovered feet are a sign of the erotic (and the beautiful) but also of the potential for infection.[22]

It is not that fully nude bodies are missing from the world of the public health posters. The nude bodies of lesbians, for example, are included in the image of the eroticized body. In a poster from the Terrence Higgins Trust in Leeds, Yorkshire, two female bodies are intertwined with the motto 'Wet your appetite for safe sex'.[23] The Austrian AIDS organization has a studied series of 'art' posters representing a series of heterosexual and homosexual partners as aesthetic Others under the motto 'Protect out of love' (illus. 65). 'Love', defined as caring and protecting, is the 'natural' extension of sexuality. For the hidden message is that the use of condoms is a sign of caring and removes sexuality from its brutal, coarse, ugly and destruct-ive mode of representation. 'Sex' is, in all these erotic presentations, sublimated into other categories such as 'love', because the visual vocabulary employed is taken from the erotic vocabulary of mass advertising. One 'loves' one's partner, says the erotic image, just as one 'loves' one's jeans. The posters refuse to treat sex *as* sex, just as advertising refuses to treat commodities *as* commodities.

These images are images of holding and touching, and commodify the closeness of 'love' to justify the use of condoms. One does not hurt the thing one loves, to reverse Oscar Wilde's dictum. And one is keyed to buy the product so presented. 'Love', here represented by the unclothed body, is the eroticized body. The French condom ads, with the motto of the Ministry of Health concerning the transmission of sexually transmitted diseases, presents similar erotic scenes of male-male touching and contact, posed as erotic posters (illus. 66). In all of these images the one at risk is the partner; the risk to the self is minimized. The beautiful Other who can be corrupted, by the agency of the self, seems to stand apart from the observer. But of course this is intended quite differently. The beautiful, youthful people at risk are all projections of the idealized self, eternally healthy, youthful and safe. In reality, say the posters, you are healthy, you are beautiful and of course you want to stay that way, so of course you are going to make sure that your partner uses a condom.

The beautiful, healthy, youthful, heterosexual couple at risk from AIDS is echoed in images from a number of national contexts. The National Programme on AIDS of the Manila Department of Health in the Philippines presents a drawing of a heterosexual pair evidently out for a night on the town with a direct warning about the transmission of AIDS and condom use (illus. 67). It is the displacement of the anxiety about identifying the Other as infected that places one's own body at risk in this context. Sexuality can be dangerous, but only, it is implied, in a bad place, even if this bad 'place' is a symbolic one, as in the 'town' in the Philippines. The German AIDS-*Hilfe*, like many European AIDS organizations, warns about sex on holidays, but the 'holiday' can be a symbolic one. Here a photograph portrays a fully dressed heterosexual couple (illus. 68), with the male gazing with desire at another fully dressed woman; he is planning a 'holiday from fidelity that is the end of safety'. Here too the image evokes a dangerous space inhabited by dangerous people, who look healthy and beautiful but are not.

Risk is represented in the broadest possible way. Thus the image of the healthy, beautiful family is central to AIDS education. The AIDS-*Hilfe* presents a gender-balanced family (father, mother, one male and one female child) with the motto 'Because I love you' (illus. 69). It resonates with the message that 'Anyone can get AIDS', which forms the theme of an American poster with a photo of a wide range of individuals of various ages, social classes and genders (illus. 70). All the figures in both these posters are clothed, for this is not the place to evoke the erotic. But all the figures are 'beautiful' – no signs here of any present illness or 'disability'.

Determining the source of infection is, however, vital. If everyone is at risk, at least if all the beautiful people are, where does the danger lie?[24] You can't tell, seems to be the model, but it is clearly beyond the self. 'Does she or doesn't she?', asks the poster of the viewer looking at the portrait of a beautiful, white woman (illus. 71). This uncertainty reflects earlier images of the 'beautiful woman', as in the 1944 American poster with the motto 'She may look clean – but pick-ups, "good" time girls, prostitutes spread syphilis and gonorrhea. You can't beat the Axis if you get VD'. The audience for the VD poster was clearly the American armed services, who were understood as male. The audience for the AIDS poster, which employs the same rhetoric and the photographic image for realism, has quite a different audience, or does it? Each of the photographs is of a beautiful female – but the VD poster employs a visual vocabulary of innocence lacking in the AIDS poster.

Abstractions of the beautiful body are used when the audience is meant to make a transition from one conceptual structure to another. In the German poster from the Ministry of Health, Youth and Women (1989), an abstract female body stands at the centre, a partial abstraction of the male cropped to one side (illus. 72). This pattern follows a radical restructuring of the image of the disease during the late 1980s from being understood as a 'gay' disease to being a disease that will affect all groups. Indeed, the abstraction of 'woman' was the means by which this restructuring was introduced, as in the Australian Federation of AIDS Organizations poster – 'The AIDS puzzle: Where do women fit?' – with an abstract image of the female body at its centre (illus. 73).[25] In the German image two young heterosexual pairs provide 'information' about the illness: 'What is AIDS?' and 'How does one acquire AIDS?'. No one mentions condom use. The narrative here is one of intrusion and insertion. No one is safe, for even 'the tiniest wound is a path for the virus to find its way into the body'. Beauty is now on a microscopic level. And visible beauty is no longer any protection. For the lesions that mark one as at risk are so minute that they cannot be seen on the body.[26]

The Body with HIV

The image of the person with HIV or active AIDS is equally beautiful. In the photographic work of Ingo Taubhorn, identical portraits of the same individuals are labelled 'I am positive' and 'I am negative' to stress the observer's inability to tell which image is HIV-positive.[27] Here the notion of 'not being able to tell' seems to be separate from the desire to protect the innocent (and beautiful) self. Rather, the argument is that people who are HIV-positive are 'not ill' as a category and are therefore 'beautiful'. But it is also clear that these images shy away from the erotic completely. The classic image is a photograph of an African-American female infant in an Urban League poster, seemingly healthy, who is represented as having 'her father's eyes and her mother's AIDS'. Accompanying this image is the warning 'Before you get pregnant, find out if you need to be tested' (illus. 74). The message is complex – the seemingly healthy baby who replicates her mother's illness, an illness with which the mother could have threatened the father, but whose end effect is on her offspring and the future of the extended group. For the seemingly healthy baby will wither and die from her mother's indiscretions, like Nana's child. A parallel image is to be found on a poster aimed at Native Americans (illus. 75), a male and female in silhouette with the motto 'Love carefully – Preserve your heritage – Know your partner!'. The elegance of the image, especially the complex lettering of the word 'LOVE', points to the preservation of the 'race'. The 'love' implied is sex, but it is extended to the image of preserving the group. This too is the message of the Boston AIDS Action Committee's recycling of the Norman Rockwell image of the father telling his son the 'facts of life' (illus. 76). The original subtext of this image, inscribed in the painting by the title of the volume held on the father's knee (*The Facts of Life*) was sexual reproduction. This is made manifest by the cat and the two kittens who frame the man and the boy, the cat associated visually with the father, the two kittens with the son. The new meaning of this image, supplied by its recontextualization by the poster, is 'Don't forget the chapter on AIDS. AIDS is a fact of life. So make sure your children get all the facts'. It is the risk to the group through the risk to the child that is stressed. Here the analogy can be made to a wide range of anti-VD posters from the early twentieth century which warned against the infection of the female because of its effect on the 'race'. The French image of the weeping mother clutching the tiny casket of her child with the motto 'Syphilis: Hereditary Illness Kills the Race' was produced for turn-of-the-century women by the Women's Education Committee of the French Society for Health and Moral Prophylaxis (illus. 29).

But the warning on the poster with the beautiful baby is that you should 'find out if you need to get tested' prior to conception. This places the burden two steps prior to conception: you must uncover if you are at risk; you must get tested; then – only if you are negative – you may conceive and bear a healthy child. Such an appeal presumes that women are self-aware, and the agents of their lives, questionable in the conservative 1980s when to bear or not bear a child was not a choice for women of all classes. What would happen if you were positive and pregnant? You would not for certain have (or be able to have) an abortion; you might rather bear an HIV-positive child. In iconographic tradition, a single sexual act by an unmarried woman necessarily results in her pregnancy, infanticide and suicide, as with Faust's Gretchen. The moral here is that bad women kill children. Similarly, a poster from the Department of Health of the City of New Orleans presents a pregnant woman and a man weeping, with the motto 'Think about it

. . . before it's too late'. Both look healthy, but the clear implication is that the future baby is at risk of infection. The mask of beauty hides the mother's corruption of her own children.

The question of race and beauty is evoked in the image of the positive individual in a poster produced by the Urban League. The drawing presents literally a bi-racial, split-screen image of weeping women, one half African-American, the other half 'white', with the implication that they are HIV-positive (illus. 77). Both halves of the image, the African-American and the 'white' halves, are represented as strikingly attractive. Likewise, a photograph from the Health Education Resource Organization in Maryland of a young and beautiful African-American couple adorns a poster with the motto 'We didn't think we could get AIDS!' (illus. 78). Here the danger is hidden within the image of the beautiful body. The need is to save the body of the HIV-infected individual as one unmarked by illness. An American poster for the Health Information Network from the early 1990s presents a seemingly healthy, middle-aged male with the motto 'In 1985, I found out I was HIV-positive. I thought it was over'. Here the implication is that the 'I' can still have a functional and erotic life even though HIV-positive, and that fact is written on my face and body. Do not take the beautiful body of even someone you are attracted to as a safe body, warn these images.

The body of the person with AIDS, like that of the healthy person at risk or the person with HIV infection, is unmarked by the signs and symptoms of the disease (Karposi's sarcoma, emaciation). In a German AIDS-*Hilfe* poster, for example, a 'healthy' woman leans over a smiling, seemingly healthy man in a hospital bed in a succouring posture. The motto of the poster is 'The Ill also Belong: Don't Give AIDS a Chance, Live Together'. Illness is represented by the context and by the new role the woman plays – no longer the potential source of illness but the mothering female as nurse. This is a standard device when the ill body is evoked. The setting or some other external sign, rather than the ill person's body, is used to evoke the disease. When the body of the person with AIDS is represented, it is always socially marked, but not physically. In a Virginia Department of Health poster the theme of the person with AIDS as melancholic/depressive (which I examined in the mid-1980s in my popular representation of the person with AIDS[28]) reappears in a public health context (illus. 79). The male body of the person with AIDS becomes that of the depressive, with all of the stigmata of isolation asssociated with this category of mental illness. Here the signs and symptoms of another stigmatized illness are used to evoke the passivity of the observer. The motto of this poster is directed at the 'healthy observer': 'It won't kill you to spend time with a friend who has AIDS'. It is the exogenous depression of isolation that marks the PWA and its cause is his social isolation. Passivity, a symptom of depression, causes the depression of the PWA through social isolation. The answer to this social isolation is also provided. In the Australian Community Support Network the person with AIDS vanishes as the focus. A smiling young man is portrayed with the motto 'Steve did something about AIDS today. Steve cooked an apple pie'. Here the person with AIDS is the object of attention but is unseen. But the symptom, the social isolation of the PWA, is presented as a curable phenomenon. Its cure is the healthy, beautiful young man carrying an apple pie.

A proof-text for our various models of reading can be found in the two 'narrative' posters that represent the entire course of AIDS in one person. The first poster was developed by the Commonwealth Department of Community Services and Health, NACAIDS, and the Aboriginal Health Workers of Australia (Queensland). Queensland is the state in Australia where the tensions between the 'white' and 'aboriginal' inhabitants are the most strained. Headed 'You don't have to be a Queenie to get AIDS: An AIDS story', this comic-strip poster (illus. 80) uses the image of the beautiful male, represented here by the sports hero, who has sex with 'someone who has AIDS', represented as a prostitute in a bar, and who returns home and infects his pregnant wife. Here an unsafe person, the prostitute, in an unsafe place, the bar, marks the origin of the illness. Heterosexual transmission takes place even to someone who is marked as robust. The transmission to the pregnant wife is implied by her melancholic expression as well as her position, head bowed, her hand on her abdomen. Here the infection of the extended group is implied with the caption 'They all get very, very sick'. For the 'all' implies not only the individuals but the clan, visualized in the hospital ward. Thus the destruction of the aboriginal people is the result of their inability to measure their own risk. It has little to do with the introduction of a wide range of other illnesses, such as tuberculosis, into their world by the 'white' Australians.

The aboriginal male is represented in the ward as dying of AIDS, his face clearly marked by the disease as he lies in bed with an HIV tube in his arm. In the world of the poster, his dying is the death of an entire people, because of the actions of even the best of them. The final panel shows the graveyard with crosses that spell out AIDS. Between the crosses are the ritual aboriginal clubs associated with masculine status. Here the attempt to distance the disease from the world of gay identity employs the 'healthy' (here meaning beautiful and heterosexual).

The second poster is from Vienna (illus. 81). Unlike the Australian poster it uses visual 'irony' to stress the course of illness. Here the tradition of the beefcake image of the male at risk is linked expressly with images of race and images of the outcome of illness. The poster employs a series of images otherwise completely taboo in the tradition of the public health poster. The beefcake images on the left side of the poster, with all its versions of safe sex, are paralleled by two inter-racial couples on the right. The stress on the extraordinarily long penis of the African (wearing a white condom) and contrasted with the small member of his partner (wearing a black condom) as well as the visible member of the Native American evokes the myths of the hypersexuality of the Other. Here the parallel to the Australian poster is evident. True danger lies in the exotic. The poster, however, not only works on a left–right opposition, but even more strikingly to underwrite this dichotomy of the place in which danger lies in terms of the upper-left and lower-right corners of the poster. The upper-right corner represents two males who use condoms, the lower-left, in clear association with the images of race, two highly disfigured males who don't use them! The passage from beauty to ugliness via the world of racial images underlines the danger – not of homosexuality – but of crossing specific cultural borders without correct defensive measures. Masculinity is shown to be at risk, but also male beauty.

In these two posters the marked body is present. The marked body places the blame, which is what all the other public health posters we have so far examined refuse to do. It localizes the blame within the victim, which is, of course, precisely the rhetoric that has been applied to AIDS in the general culture – people with AIDS 'brought it upon themselves'. But it also associates this blame with images of racial difference and with the question of the narratives imposed on those who are represented as different.

Death and Dying in the Imagery of AIDS

The Australian poster with its representation of dying also works because of the medium selected. The comic strip tells a story. There is a clear lesson to be learned from it; a lesson of fidelity and the avoidance of risk. But this story only works in its detailed representation of the dying body because in the world of the comic, an unreal world on the very margins of reality, choices can have immediate consequences and every negative act adequate punishment. Here the effect is on the group, itself afraid of vanishing under the onslaught of European culture, its attractions, and its dangers.

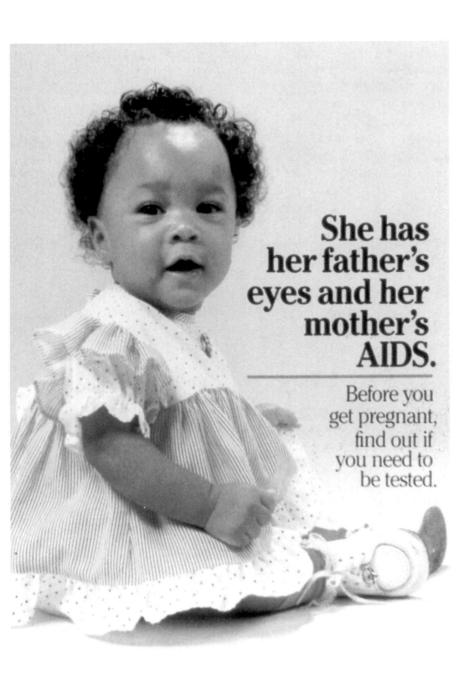

Before you get pregnant, find out if you need to be tested.

74 A poster from the Urban League, one of the oldest African-American organizations, representing the danger that lies beneath the skin, even that of a child.

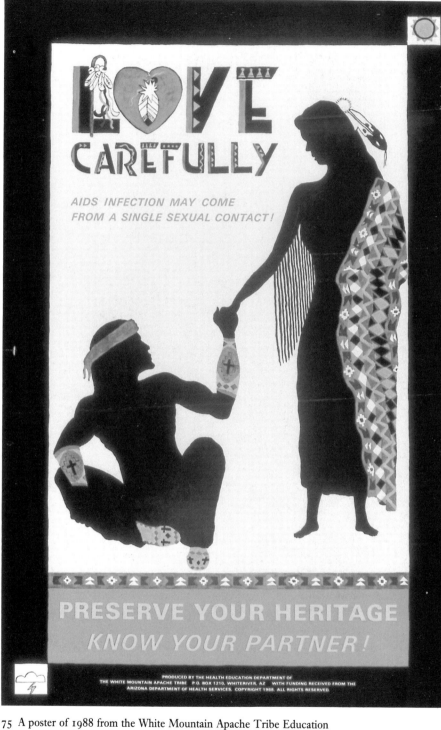

75 A poster of 1988 from the White Mountain Apache Tribe Education Department in Arizona.

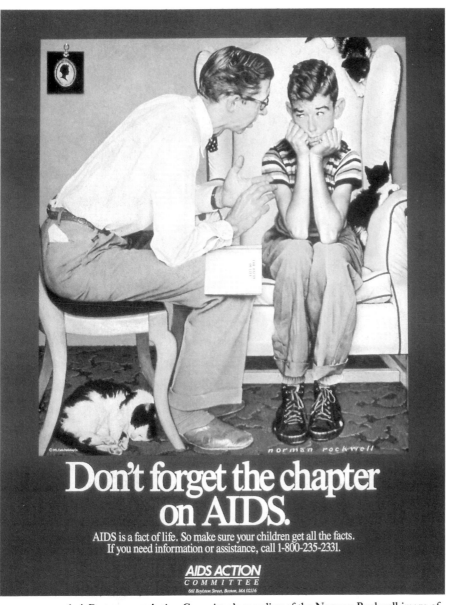

Don't forget the chapter on AIDS.

AIDS is a fact of life. So make sure your children get all the facts.
If you need information or assistance, call 1-800-235-2331.

AIDS ACTION
COMMITTEE
661 Boylston Street, Boston, MA 02116

76 A Boston AIDS Action Committee's recycling of the Norman Rockwell image of the father telling his son about the 'facts of life'.

YOU CAN GET AIDS

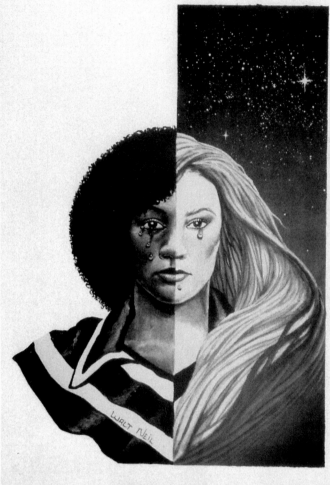

For Information About
AIDS Contact

The Urban League

or call 1-800-332-AIDS

AIDS Does Not Discriminate

77 The composite person with AIDS is black and white, rather than male and female, in this poster from the Urban League.

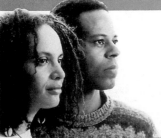

"We Didn't Think We Could Get AIDS!"

50% of the cases of AIDS
in Maryland are black.

The best defense against AIDS is information.

Call **HERO**
Health Education Resource Organization

945-AIDS • 251-1164 • 1-800-638-6252
Baltimore Metro   DC Metro   Elsewhere in MD

'HERO 1987

78 A Health Education Resource Organization, Maryland, poster of 1987 showing a young and beautiful African American couple.

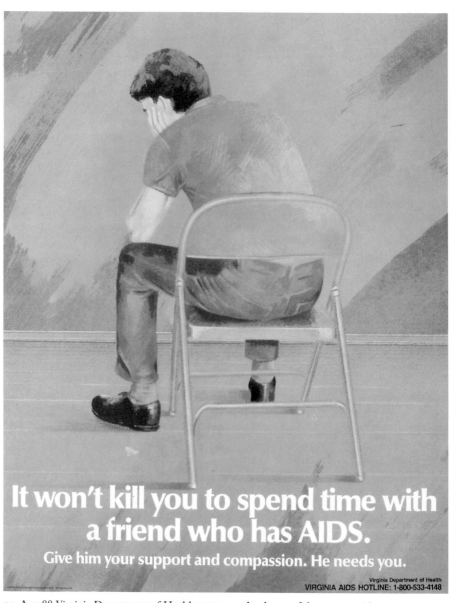

It won't kill you to spend time with a friend who has AIDS.

Give him your support and compassion. He needs you.

Virginia Department of Health
VIRGINIA AIDS HOTLINE: 1-800-533-4148

79 A 1988 Virginia Department of Health poster on the theme of the person with AIDS as melancholic/depressive. Melancholy also reflects the social isolation associated with the popular image of the person with AIDS.

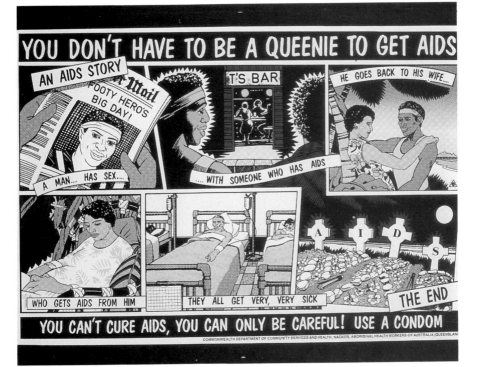

80 A narrative poster from the Commonwealth Department of Community Services and Health, 'NACAIDS' [National Advisory Committee on AIDS] and the Aboriginal Health Workers of Australia (Queensland).

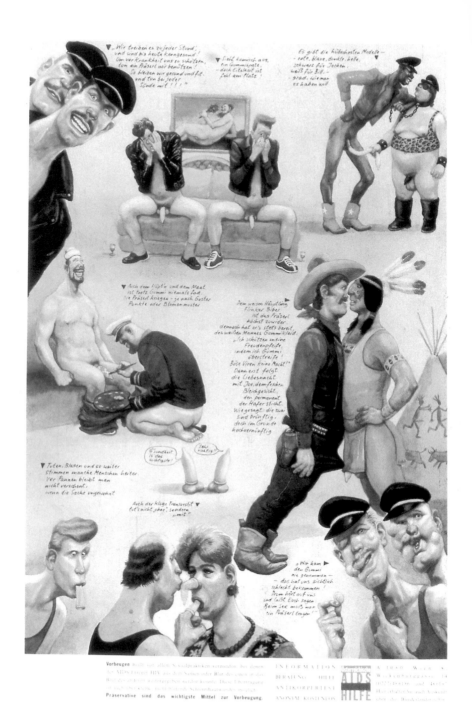

81 A narrative poster from Austria's AIDS-*Hilfe*.

Certainly the most intense counterpoint to the image of the body of the person with AIDS being represented as a 'healthy' and beautiful body is the micro-scandal around an advertisement that Benetton Mills, the Italian clothing company, released in January 1992.[29] The ad showed a photograph of an AIDS hospital deathbed scene, with a distraught man holding the dead, or dying, body of his starkly emaciated son, while a younger and an older woman comfort one other at the foot of the bed. This was not a 'public health' advertisement, but placed AIDS in the visual context of a major social (not 'natural') catastrophe. This deathbed scene was part of a six-page series of images run by Benetton in the stylish magazines *Vanity Fair* and *Vogue*, which included a car in flames and a ship swamped with desperate Albanian refugees.[30] These ads clearly intended to identify the sweater maker with social causes that it believed were important to the youthful purchasers of its woollens. (Benetton is not a maker of anything, but a consortium that moves its contracts from one Third World country to another in order to keep its labour costs low.) But the image of the person with AIDS was unique, as it called forth an immediate and hostile reaction on the part of those groups active in promoting the image of the 'beautiful' body with/at risk from AIDS. As a counter-gesture, the company (completely in line with its advertising policy), agreed to distribute a brochure on safe sex prepared by the Gay Men's Health Crisis in the July 1992 issue of *Spin* magazine. This brochure had no images of individuals dying, and maintained the image of the healthy and beautiful body.[31]

Here the question of why Benetton so misread the meaning of the representation of the body of the person dying from AIDS should be understood. It is clear that the public health discourse in the United States and Europe about AIDS in the early 1990s had stressed the risk of heterosexual transmission over all other problems. Youthful purchasers, it could be assumed, would have defined their own well-being against the notion of risk (from fire, war, the collapse of governments, disease). Our beautiful bodies, this discourse ran, are permanent and unmarred despite all the risks present in the world. And we are even more secure – and cuddly – in woollen sweaters. But what the observer desired, especially the gay observer confronted with the photograph, was the unmarked erotic body of the PWA at the moment of death. With the actual photograph of the body dying, no safe-sex eroticism could separate the body at risk from the moment of death – a universal human anxiety about death. Even the parent's protection cannot shield the individual from the reality of death. To trespass even visually on the reality of death would have violated an American compact.

It is not that death is missing from the vocabulary of the public health posters. Death is present, but dying is missing or mediated by genre expectations, as in the Australian poster discussed above. The stark realism of the Benetton advertisement seems to be an impossibility for public health announcements in an age in which the culture is full of images of dying and loss.[32] Central to all these public health posters is the notion that the erotic and AIDS are linked in the sphere of the beautiful. Only death is ugly, but it is an ugliness mediated by employing a historical icon. The image of death in these posters is that of the classical *memento mori*. The image of the skeleton as the symbol of the body unshrouded by its eroticized layer of skin, the skin which reveals every truth and every disease, is a classical trope.[33] Such images, as in the late eighteenth-century work of Jacques Gamelin, preserve a certain distance from the act of dying; indeed, they evoke the symbolic potential of the resurrection. Often, a contrasting image of the 'healthy' body is presented in these images as a contrast to the *memento mori*. This again is a traditional juxtaposition, as in Hans Baldung's *Eve, the Serpent and Death* (1515), which reveals the 'skeleton beneath the skin', the inevitability of death lurking beneath the erotic surface. The erotic, and in Eve's case, the seductive, is revealed to be but a mask for disease and death, not only for the individual but for all human beings. All this is represented for the viewer by seeing the act of touching. The viewer is shielded from danger (because the viewer only looks) while watching that most dangerous of acts, the act of touching.

In the world of the public health poster, this polluting touch is evoked in the images of AIDS associated with the dangers attendant on HIV drug-users in sharing used needles. Here an entirely new vocabulary is introduced that should be free from any sexual overtones. But the symbolic representation of the penetration of the body evokes much the same fear of pollution as do all forms of sexual penetration. The bounds of the polluting touch, even within the context of medical treatment, echo the general cultural association of AIDS and touch. In a 1987 British public health poster entitled 'Heads you live. Tails you get AIDS', a disembodied hand reaches out to offer us a filled hypodermic (illus. 82). The dark background is covered in blood. The message is clear – here is the deathly touch, the polluting power of blood. In American culture during the early 1990s this association was power-fully made in the cinema. Francis Ford Coppola's film *Bram Stoker's Dracula* (1992) associates blood (as seen through a microscope) and the markings on the neck of the vampire's victims to evoke the visual vocabulary of AIDS with its images of blood, skin cancer, and death.[34] But here it is not the *pars par toto* which is sought – for Coppola stressed the complete transformation of the body and character of the infected person. In these posters the blood (rather than the sexual fluids, such as semen, which are often mentioned but never, never represented in any of these posters) serves as the locus of the disease outside of the body. The analogy with the posters that stressed the sexual transmission of AIDS is clear – the dirty needle is the dirty (read ugly) penis, while the blood is the semen (or vaginal fluid). And the needles are always poised in readiness, like the erect penises represented in some of the posters, at the very moment of infiltration. But here no eroticism mediates the risk.

The symbolic figure of Death, as in the classic image of the Grim Reaper, comes to represent the touch of the dirty needle. This motif repeats itself again and again. In an image from the National Advisory Committee on AIDS from the late 1980s (illus. 83), the caption is 'AIDS. Sharing needles is just asking for it'. There the skeletal hand of Death personified, draped in a shroud, offers a 'healthy' hand a full hypodermic needle. In a parallel image from a poster entitled 'Dead Give Away' the same theme is repeated (illus. 84). Death and drugs seem a linked concept. The New York City Department of Health provides an image of the Grim Reaper playing cards, juxtaposed with a healthy hand, holding cards marked A, I, D and S and the motto 'Don't let AIDS deal you a losing hand. Know the facts: Don't shoot drugs or share needles' (illus. 85). The Multicultural AIDS Needle Users Project in San Francisco evokes the image of the 'stacked deck' with the image of the Death's-head and the motto 'Don't gamble with AIDS . . . it's a stacked deck' in a poster teaching how to clean needles with bleach (illus. 86). Over and over, the hand, the icon of touch, comes to stand for the potentially deadly touch, just as the erotic touch has hidden within it the potential for pain. And this is evoked precisely in the piercing and painful touch used in a poster from 1989 that incorporated a painting of the martyrdom of St Sebastian by the seventeenth-century Piedmontese artist Tanzio da Varallo (illus. 87). It is the painful sexualized touch that is evoked here with the image of St Sebastian, an image that has wide currency in the gay community. Death as the symbolic representation of the effect of the polluting touch is, however, not solely employed to represent the overtly non-erotic activity of taking HIV drugs.

The image of Death comes to be used as a marker for the effect of the disease irrespective of its origin. The Urban League in the United States employs a contrasting image of an evidently 'healthy' mother and her 'healthy' baby encased in a skull whose upper jaw spells AIDS with the motto 'You can get AIDS' (illus. 88). And this image of AIDS and Death is not to be found merely within the American context. The Ministry of Health in Brunei provides an image of a skull and the bilingual motto 'AIDS? Protect yourself by knowing about it' (illus. 89). In a Nigerian poster from the Federal Ministry of Health in Lagos, the possibilities of acquiring the disease are tabulated. One of them, sexual contact, is represented by two 'beautiful' men and a woman who are presented with a skull in their midst and the motto 'Sexual Contact with an Infected Person'. The person with HIV suddenly becomes, like the person who wishes to share his/her 'works' with you, Death personified.

Rarely is the figure of Death as an abstraction replaced by representations (even symbolic representations) of a dead body. The final images of Death are the only ones that employ a non-symbolic image, for example a photograph of a shrouded body on a trolley, its feet exposed and presented to the audience in the manner of Mantegna's Christ, and labelled 'Don't let love sweep you off your feet' (illus. 90). An equivalent Spanish-language poster exists with a sketch of the same scene, a body-tag on the toe, with only the feet exposed and the motto 'The risk is of death' (illus. 91). Here the body is not only dead but shrouded, an anonymous figure separate from the cares and anxieties of the living. AIDS comes to be associated with Death, but not with the process of dying. The anonymity of public death, unlike the caring dying represented in the Benetton advertisement, marks the bad death, the solitary death, the death that ends up in a public morgue.

The image of the 'positive' body or the body with AIDS is strictly controlled in the world of the public health poster. Nowhere is an image of the 'ugly' or diseased body evoked directly, for any such evocation would refer back to the initial sense of AIDS as a 'gay' disease and the powerful effect this has had on the re-pathologization of homosexuality. *Mens non sana in corpore insano* cannot be the motto. For representing the ill body as a dying body is not possible. Such a body would point to 'deviance from the norm' in the form of illness. And this association with homosexuality and addiction labelled as illness must be suppressed. The 'beautiful' remains the transnational sign for the healthy and the 'ugly' is banished from this world of images. Yet hidden within the images of the beautiful is the potential for death. Death comes to be limited as the beautiful body moves to its antithesis without the processes of dying. Death itself comes to be aestheticized. All these images are images not of education, but of control. They seek to present worlds that are as static as the images themselves. The dynamic reality of dying as part of the life-cycle and its real, concrete, frightening presence for those stricken with AIDS is denied and repressed. When we view these posters, we are educated in the potential for action – which is what advertising does best, but little else. The chimerical world of picturing beauty and health at the close of the twentieth century provides as little access to the complex images demanded of our society as do the images of the last *fin de siècle*, but in their overwhelming simplicity they form the materials for a new history of medicine rooted in the study of the visual image.

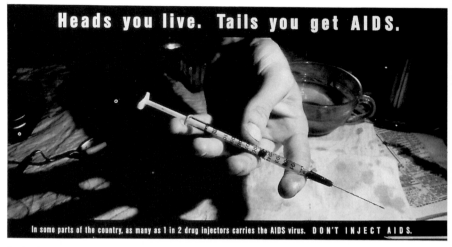

82 In this British public health poster of 1987 a disembodied hand reaches out as if to offer us a filled hypodermic.

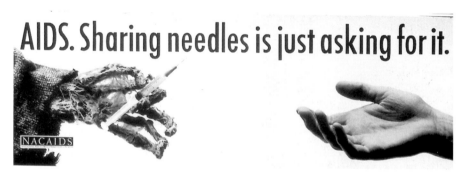

83 The *memento mori* as the image of the painful, infectious touch of the dirty needle is evoked in this 'NACAIDS' poster from the late 1980s.

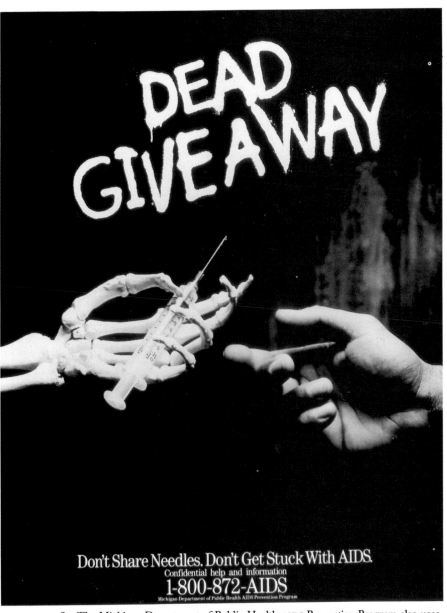

DEAD GIVEAWAY

Don't Share Needles. Don't Get Stuck With AIDS.
Confidential help and information
1-800-872-AIDS
Michigan Department of Public Health AIDS Prevention Program

84 The Michigan Department of Public Health AIDS Prevention Program also uses the *memento mori* in the context of the polluting touch of the needle.

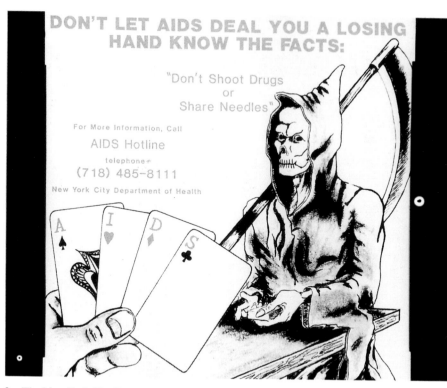

85 The New York City Department of Health employs the 'Grim Reaper' as a warning against intravenous drug use.

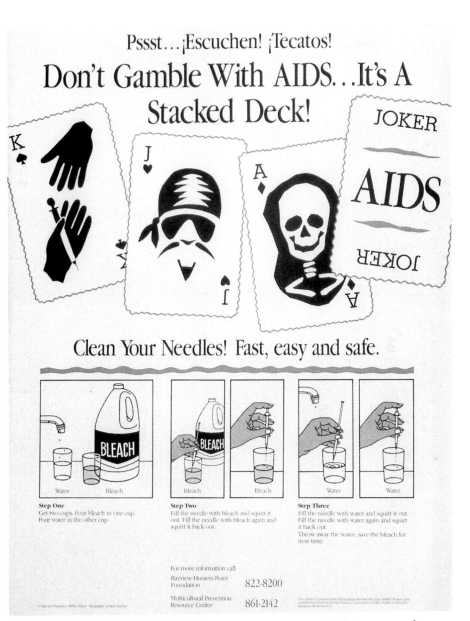

86 'Pssst . . . ! Listen! Watch out!'. The rules that would help intravenous drug users avoid HIV infection are spelt out in this poster using a death's-head, from the San Francisco Multicultural AIDS Needle Users Project.

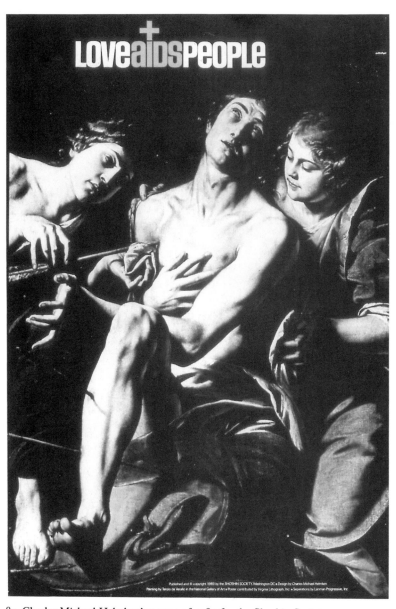

87 Charles Michael Helmken's poster of 1989 for the Shoshin Society
incorporating Tanzio da Varallo's 17th-century *Martyrdom of St Sebastian* (in the
National Gallery of Art, Washington), echoing the implication of the dangerous
touch of sexually transmitted disease. The dangerous touch encompasses all the
anxiety about entering the body, including the syringe entering the body of the drug
abuser. Here the arrows serve multiple symbolic purposes.

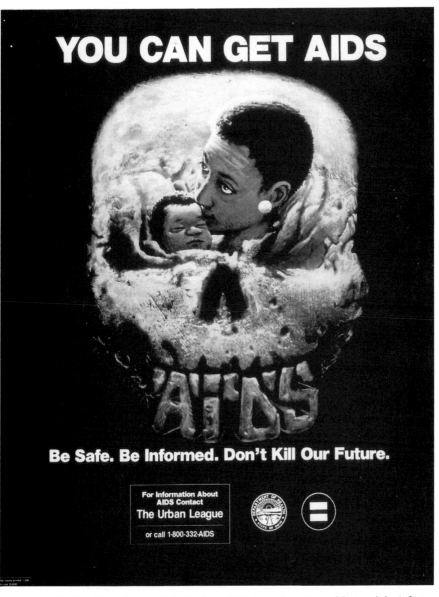

88 The Urban League links the beautiful baby and mother as Mary and the infant Jesus in a quasi-religious image of the *memento mori*.

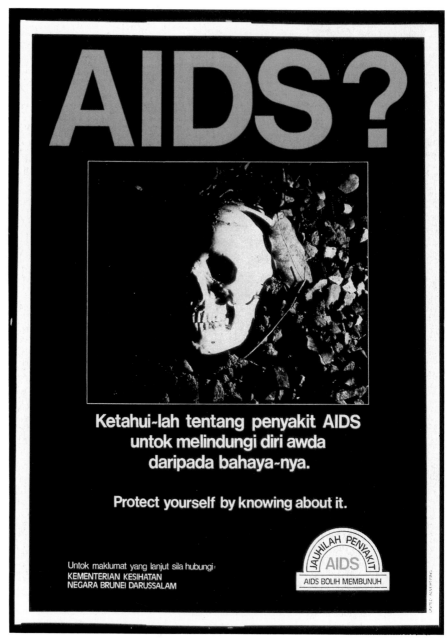

89 'AIDS? Know what AIDS is in order to protect yourself from it. . . . You must avoid AIDS because it is fatal. Protect yourself by knowing about it': The Ministry of Health in Brunei provides an image of a skull and dried leaves symbolising death.

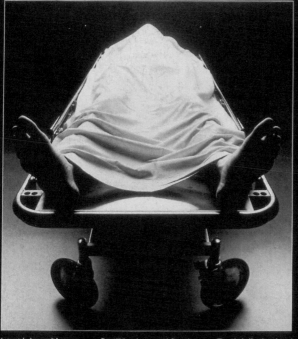

DON'T LET LOVE SWEEP YOU OFF YOUR FEET.

Unfortunately, love won't keep you from getting AIDS. Sleep with the wrong person and you may wake up to the hard cold facts about AIDS too late.

Because when you sleep with someone, you're sleeping with everyone he or she has slept with for the past eight years.

And there's no known cure for AIDS. Everyone who gets the disease dies.

But AIDS can be prevented. By saying no to sex. And by saying no to needle drugs.

Sure, sex can be embarrassing to talk about, but don't let it embarrass you to death. Get all the facts about AIDS, and talk about them with your girlfriend or boyfriend.

Then if you choose to have sex, stick to one partner. And always use a condom. It's one of the best defenses against AIDS.

The point is, if you're going to have sex, you should do it responsibly.

So don't take AIDS lying down. For more information on how AIDS is transmitted and how you can protect yourself. Call the Dallas County Health Department, (214) 351-4335. All calls are confidential.

AIDS. IT CAN'T BE CURED. BUT IT CAN BE PREVENTED.

90 Religious imagery becomes alienated and secularized as the feet of Christ become the image of the feet of the person dead with AIDS in this poster from Dallas, Texas.

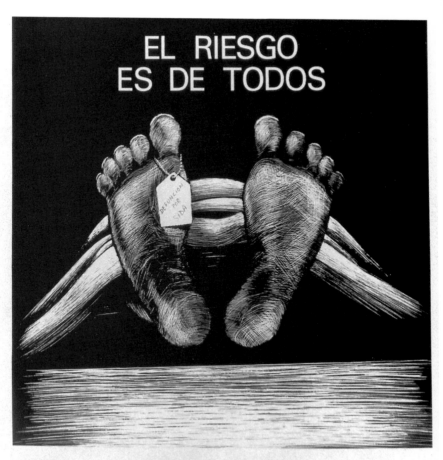

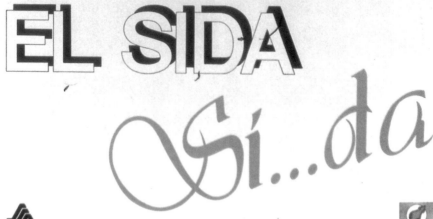

91 'The risk is of death': This Spanish-language poster from Conasida [SIDA = AIDS] in New York evokes a similar use of the secularized religious imagery of death, perhaps also drawing on Mantegna's famous depiction of the dead Christ.

Towards a Conclusion

This book provides a series of historical narratives on the relationship between health and disease, beauty and ugliness. It does not make any claims for comprehensiveness, either in its coverage of this question or in the totality of its reading of the texts and images offered. They are *readings* – from the end of the millennium, seen from the perspective of a Jewish-American academic in the post-Shoah age of AIDS. My readings make no claim to being exhaustive interpretations in any sense; I am not attempting to give the only (perhaps not even the best) examinations, but only my present take on each of these manifestations. My readings of the images in this book are framed through my understanding of the complexity of the historical settings I have reconstructed. They too have to be partial, incomplete, though they are rooted in an analysis of the discourses of the distant or near past.

Thus I provide few answers to the complex questions raised about the relationship between the realms of the aesthetic and the pathological. Rather, these foregoing chapters are attempts to frame a series of questions that seem important to me in my time in ways that seem to make sense to me. I would hope that others would enter into my vision of this material, enabling them to share with me my sense of the importance of this question at the close of the twentieth century. The narratives I offer are my own stories based on my reading and viewing of cultural artefacts, but the images are also provided for the reader's analysis. Such a book could be read ('looked at') without my analysis, since the very selection and ordering of the images provides a parallel narrative to my text. Thus the images are also anecdotal. And all my tales reflect my understanding of the function of such studies. My narratives and images have 'mimetic' value, not by reflecting some fancied set of rigid facts about the world, but by cataloguing the cultural fantasies of that world as made concrete within the world of images.

The pictures in this book are thus to be read neither as 'merely' illustrations or even as 'merely' visual sources. They should be seen as the proof texts for the central problem of this book, the easy association between the beautiful and the healthy, the ugly and the ill, and the inscription of these analogies into the medical and aesthetic cultures of the West. At the end of the twentieth century we live – perhaps more than ever before – in an age of the image in all of its complexity. And this becomes more evident at the moment of the decline of one of its means of the mechanical reproduction of images, the illustrated medical book. It seems to be true, as I intimated in the opening chapter, that the history of the illustrated medical book in the age of mechanical reproduction that began in the fifteenth century may be drawing to a close today. Studying such still images of illness while excluding moving images at the close of the twentieth century has been problematic. This has been true especially given the special significance attached to the still image in the world of medicine, such as its claim on mimesis in a world where moving images make even greater claims on representing the 'real' world of the body. Medical textbooks, for example, use pictures to provide substitutes for 'real' patients or 'real' specimens. These images are given the aura of 'reality' in this context. Yet all of these claims for the truthfulness of these images are rooted in the aesthetics of the body, aesthetics that associate beauty, health, truthfulness and morality in opposition to ugliness, illness, falsity and immorality.

Working on the history of still images from and about the world of medicine has had its own rationale. Still images of health and illness have even an older history than that of the printed book. This history provides an unreflected record of the fantasies about the body, its illnesses and their representation. They also reflect the quality of the aesthetic as well as the mimetic that has been associated with the world of the still image. But at the end of the twentieth century the world of medicine employs moving images of all types as a matter of course. New CD-ROM packages from the world of medicine and the teaching of medicine permit the most complex combination of static images, moving image and text in an interactive manner. More complex than medical films, such CD-ROM textbooks provide a complex model for a new 'reality' of health and disease and its relationship to the new aesthetics of cyberspace and hyperreality. No longer can one simply look at the static image as the best reflection of the world of medical image-making.

Indeed, even the historiography of static medical images has begun to change because of this new technology. Huge video-discs of medical images from the Wellcome Institute (London) and the National Library of Medicine (Bethesda, Maryland) enable a type of sorting and contrast impossible in the past. Their complex databases make the demand on the historian studying static images quite different. The simple cataloguing of visual analogies (such as 'the image of the tubercular in medicine') is no longer of interest once such analogies can be generated by software. Analysis rather than tabulation must be the goal of the historian of medicine using still images. And that analysis must reflect the complexity of the role that static images play in the world of moving images. Such analysis should be anecdotal at this stage. For comprehensive studies of images are indeed but extended catalogues. Framing each image from the specific standpoint of the historian–viewer (as I have done in this book) provides the potential for each viewer to generate the context that will supply the most meaningful narrative for him or her. Each context must be rooted in the discourses of the time (both that of the object and that of the viewer), but the selection and stress of the narrative is determined by the needs and interest of the narrator.[1]

The purpose of the selective (rather than the statistical or exhaustive) study of images of health and disease, especially in regard to patterns of textual contextualization, is to enable the reader to enter into the process of analysis. The anecdotal and the incidental have become permissible methods of studying culture in our day and age. But this is especially true of still images. Unlike studies of the novel or film, the reader 'sees' the object in a relatively unmediated manner. The still image is reproduced on the page and is not reduced to my retelling of the plot line or of a formal, shot-by shot narration of the film. While it is true that the image may be ripped from the context of the illustrated book, in some cases I have even supplied the full page of the book to provide some further contextualization. The reader/viewer of this volume can engage with me about the images that I reproduce and the tales that I tell about them.

Here we have a very modern project – the telling of multiple tales about a single object – that reveals some of the permanence of the anxieties of our age in regard to the body and to the memory of the body from the past.[2] While we recognize the potential for such multiple tales, we still struggle to find one that is 'true'. For flux is disturbing, permanence reassuring, even in the telling of stories. The ultimate flux that is combated in our telling of stories is that flux experienced in our sensing the transience of our lives and bodies. This is the reason we compulsively tell tales about health and illness; it is in these tales that we come closest to articulating the anxieties we have about our own mortality. These tales are as much present in the culture of medicine as in that of art.

Living and dying are the models of all art and all culture; these moments of hope and despair frame who we are and what we fear we must become. The anxiety about multiple, simultaneous readings with their potential to reveal the absence of any permanence is but a reflection of our inherent anxiety about the transience of our control over ourselves and our world. But it is not birth and death but living and dying that we struggle to understand, that we must control through our world of representations. As Cornelius Castoriadis showed two decades ago, the imaginary constructs of society provide the space in which these fearful, ever shifting boundaries are exorcized. Our social and cultural construction of the ideas of the beautiful and of ugliness are ways of controlling this slipperiness in the world of culture. Given that, as Ernesto Laclau and Chantal Mouffe have argued, every society strives to create the illusion of internal harmony, it is no surprise that within the cultural realms, such as the worlds of medicine and the aesthetic that determine the very fabric of 'society', this desire for control is also present. Slavoj Žižek has more recently seen that there is an ongoing, dialectical relationship between this desire for a seamless world (that masks the slipperiness of reality) and the impossibility of truly comprehending our position in that ever-changing world. Žižek mirrors Lacan's view that we see fantasy as a defence against the open question 'che vuoi?' (What do you want?). It is this unspoken question that clearly frames the field of the cultural imaginary. Through the symbolic order (here understood as aesthetics or medicine or the aesthetics of medicine) we can have the illusion of bridging the gap between our need to sense ourselves as immutable individuals and our anxiety about our own mutability. What do you want? A sense of the boundaries of the self. The ideas of the aesthetic remain cultural constructs in the imaginary, but they are also projected into the world and form our perception of the individuals about us and their perception of themselves. They are a means of controlling (or at least delimiting) the Other. The beautiful and the ugly thus become seemingly permanent markers that evoke other such boundaries (truth/fiction; health/disease). In the cultural imaginary these function as 'real' borders that cannot be transgressed precisely because they are arbitrary divisions that need to be constantly reinforced.[3]

All of these narratives of aesthetics and pathology deal with power, but it is not solely power generated by social tension. It is also a sense of loss and the illusion of control to be found within the imaginary. It is there that resistance can take place with greater ease than in the social world of institutions and human interactions. It is there that the symbolic dominates and translates lived and fantasized experience into the complex meaning represented by the image. James Hillman has observed that the 'image is always more complex than the concept'.[4] It is also so much more complex than the 'day residue' that is the trace of power in our fantasies about the world.

It is in the image, then, that the memory of desire, the desire for permanence and stability, is best preserved. It is these memories, faint and obscure, that have their origin in our initial anxiety about ourselves as separate and distinct in the world. The image and its symbolic language can be the space where the memories of trauma are articulated – or it can be the site of their most radical repression. The image can be mausoleum or memorial, the spur of memory or its mummification. The image can serve as the visual, symbolic memory of a culture but also be the seat of its most violent suppressions. Each age builds its monuments to memory and calls them art. They seem to be solid and permanent and, indeed, we need them to appear so. The seeming solidity of the image, however, is constantly undermined by our ability to reinterpret, to change, to alter it through our acts of remembering.

Thus the visual image also provides a space for the working through of contradictory experiences not represented in monuments. Seeking the 'truth' in art means seeking after the expression of the trace memories of the past and their expression in a new and as yet unstable sense of the present. Such memories are not yet articulated, not yet formed, yet always present in the world of the visual. The image contains much more than the concept because it is the field in which the memory of the first trauma, our initial sense of our separateness from the world, can be recast and reworked.

The anxiety of becoming one in the world is accompanied always by the sense of loss. It is in the image – whether the image from high art or from the world of medicine – that the loss is best captured. It is not at all the simple claim of the primacy of vision. In the past 500 years (since the introduction of printing) the claim to the primacy of the visual has forced us to repress its complex reduction of reality to that most 'rational' of senses – sight. The very idea of the image thus also contains within it a series of repressed memories. In the West we have made the claim that rationality and sight are inexorably linked and have relegated other senses (especially touch and smell/taste) to the realm of the lower senses, of the irrational.[5] In doing so, we have repressed their presence in the world of the imaginary and have spoken about our dreams and our dreaming as only a world of sight symbolized. The image of the body represented in this book, however, also evokes the touch of the body and its smell. Disease is not solely *seen* in the Other;

its 'stench' fills our nostrils and floods our imagination. It does not respect the nice clean boundary that we have attributed to the sense of sight. Our eyes register; our noses inhale; our fingers stroke. We smell ourselves and others and yet repress that aspect of the world as too primitive, too crude, too close to ourselves. And the sense of touch is also banned. We are constantly in 'touch' with our own bodies and those of others. Touch permeates our sense of self – waking and sleeping – and reinforces the particular normality that we sense when we do not sense our bodies. As Nietzsche wrote, we feel our bodies only once we become ill. Our teeth, our skin, our viscera are always and constantly subconsciously felt, yet they become part of our consciousness only when they are 'diseased' and pain us. It is in the world of the imaginary that these qualities reappear and these are the qualities that are repressed in the act of seeing images.

Thus the visual image evokes both the visual symbolic and the sensory web about the healthy and diseased body that is repressed by the very act of seeing the visual image. Freud's own emphasis on the imagined visual in his construction of the dream work represses the evocation of other sensory fields in the dream. For we smell, touch and taste in our dreams, much as the muscular response of the sleeping dog indicates its kinaesthetic response to dreams (of chasing cats?). We awaken and remember the visual representation of such bits of day residue, for we are actively censoring our memories because of the meaning ascribed to and the affect associated with the 'lower' senses. In models of the symbolic language of the dream, such as condensation and visualization, the translation of one experiential model (such as smell) into another (such as sight) is the result of our superego's unconscious censoring of the power of this realm of the senses and its evocation of the most basic sense of our separateness.

When we explore the history of images, therefore, we move toward the unseen that is also present. In my discussion of noses and their loss, smell is rarely evoked. The association of the missing nose with smell, and with the stench of the rotting, syphilitic body – Nana's body putrefying on the bier at the close of Zola's novel – is ubiquitous, and yet rarely evoked in the world of images. Yet the reader sees Nana's corpse in the words on the page or in the illustrations that accompany the text. Her smell (and our nose) is evoked but not present. Our presence as readers/observers is made tolerable only through this mediation. The filter of the image enables the reader to confront even the body putrefying *before* death. The loss of the nose is accompanied by the vision of the living putrefaction of the body, by its stench. And yet the images only seem to represent the body seen, the body studied, the body distant. We experience the body as seemingly in control through the world of the visual. We censor out the association with the world of the ugly and of decay – the mark of our own decay, our own gradual collapse. For smell and touch evoke for us the world before language: they are the keys to repressed memories of the wholeness of a world not primarily seen but felt and tasted and smelt. Each time such a world is half remembered, its loss and the loss of the wholeness with that world and the control over it is also evoked. The trauma of loss reappears in the censored world of the visual imaginary.

The censorship is found not only in the turn-of-the-century world of the Opéra ghost and that of the 'grandes horizontales', such as Nana, but also in the world of AIDS. Our anxiety about our own vulnerability is present in the images of people with AIDS. AIDS inhabits our visual world at the close of the twentieth century. It is captured in images of dying, skeletal bodies, skin marked by open sores and lesions. In the West these representations of dying are remembered in the world of images in which the primary visual association is with the emaciated, distorted bodies from black-and-white news photographs of the newly liberated concentration camps in 1945. Suddenly the emaciated bodies of the people with AIDS echo those images of horror and ugliness; bodies destroyed by illness and homophobic politics just as the bodies in the camps were deformed by the politics that ascribed specific illnesses to the Jews. Mark Twain's unconscious fantasy about the ill bodies of the Jews in the Holy Land was part of the myth-making with the European and American imaginary that was eventually shaped into the quite real world of the death camps. The line from Twain's benign 'liberal' view to that of the most repulsive anti-Semitic film of the Third Reich, Fritz Hippler's *The Eternal Jew* (1940), is relatively straight if we map it onto the cultural imagination concerning the relation of the Jews to the model of health and beauty or illness and ugliness.

The world of the 1990s needed to reformat the visual memories of the victims of the Holocaust, as Steven Spielberg does in *Schindler's List* (1993). Spielberg's vision of the Holocaust resuscitates and reinvigorates the black-and-white images torn from newspapers and weekly newsreels. The cultural imaginary of AIDS is a world framed by that experience of death and dying, of isolation and stigmatization. It is not that the experience of AIDS in society is 'like' the Holocaust, nor is AIDS a new 'holocaust', but that the visual world of AIDS is framed for me by the visual memory of the Shoah and its trauma. Furthermore, it is also a set of cultural images with a history.

It is vital to understand the world of images as already pre-programmed and reused. Alain Resnais in his *Night and Fog* used footage from the liberation of the camps – pictures of emaciated, tortured bodies being pushed into pits by bulldozers – as a means of commenting on the universal potential for nuclear disaster in the 1950s. Such images were the direct answer to images from Hippler. Hippler's representation of the 'Jew' provided a visual code that transformed the Jews into the source of disease and death (like the rats that carry the plague in Hippler's analogy). Here the 'disease' ('the madness of the German leaders such as Hitler') is ascribed to the Germans and the corpses are proof of the pathological state of the leadership of the Third Reich. The move from the 'madness of the Nazis' to the 'madness of nuclear war' seemed a natural one for Resnais. But the power of all of these images lies in the association of the deformed, emaciated bodies and destroyed physiognomies with the aesthetics of illness and its reading in the West.

Thus these images have a history by the time we reach the 1980s and '90s. The images in the public health world are the antithesis of that tradition – they are the slick, polished images that are to clarify rather than generate fear about the coherence of one's own body. Fear and loathing are missing from the world of AIDS as represented in the public health representations of the body with AIDS. Not only has all smell, all touch been removed from this world – as indeed it was removed by the reduction of the experience of the Holocaust for readers and movie-goers of the 1990s to visual images, for we remember not the events but rather images of the events, stripped of everything but the visual. Such a loss is inherent to the medium of film and its absence is not overtly evident. The visual world of the Shoah is the background for my understanding of the image of the person with AIDS. Yet the visual tradition against which the public health advertisements discussed in the final chapter of this book work is the image of mass death. At the close of the century such images are the viewer's daily television fare (and even appear in advertisements for sweaters). Whether these images come from Somalia or Rwanda and appear on CNN or on the front pages of daily newspapers, they evoke 'holocausts' because of the powerful nature of the images and the context in which these images are read. So AIDS too is seen as a 'holocaust'. But here the public images are (for the most part) not analogous to the images of mass dying. They are the images of healthy bodies, unmarked bodies, while the dying continues. The stench of rotting flesh, the smell of pus, the infected sputum, the open lesions, the chronic anxiety about the body that marks the disease of AIDS in the West is effaced in our public inability to deal with the dying, a dying that can and does affect all of us.

AIDS should have a different face in Africa, where it has already become one of the major killers. Rwanda was the site of one of the great ethnic massacres of the past decade; it is also one of the worst sites for cases of AIDS in the world. Rwanda was already the site of a mass death, but one unreceived by the general viewing public in the West because of our anxiety about our own vulnerability to AIDS and the other 'new' diseases that have suddenly (re-)appeared in our back-yards: the 'new' cholera, the 'new' tuberculosis, the 'new' syphilis. Many of these diseases are as 'new' as AIDS because they have been seen as diseases of the past. Many are 'new' because they have been so changed by exposure to the specifics against them that our first-line defence, the world of drugs, is no longer completely effective. Many are 'new' because these illnesses are now read in relationship to the meaning ascribed to AIDS in Western and post-colonial societies. (Thus syphilis has been read as coterminous or identical with AIDS and tuberculosis as a disease now primarily affecting individuals with an impaired immune system. The 'new' tuberculosis, which comes to be associated in the 1990s with AIDS, evokes the debates about control, about meaning and about focus, which prove to be the means of providing a sense of the recycling of the symbolic structures associated with illness at the close of the millennium.) Yet of course these illnesses are truly not the same as their earlier counterparts: they have different contexts, and are read in different ways in the complex Western cultures in which we live, than were those or their parallels 100 years ago. But there is more than a slight sense of continuity. Part of this may well be the simple sense of repetition built into the calendar, for turns of century have a great symbolic significance in the meaning we attribute to the calendar. But there are other meanings that do transcend merely the markers of chronological time. Thus there are meanings with which we wrestled whose structure was cast 100 years ago. One can learn from the debates about the meaning of an illness even after a century. Thus the anxiety associated with the debate about compulsory reporting and hospitalization that accompanied tuberculo-sis has interesting parallels in our contemporary debates about compulsory reporting and hospitalization of people who are HIV positive. It is not the same illness, but the questions that arise, questions of the possibility of cure, of stigmatization, of family responsibility, of anxiety about the body politic, are all present in both times with both diseases.

This was brought home to me in the summer of 1994. I spent that summer teaching in South Africa – the 'new' South Africa. In Johannesburg, HIV infection and AIDS is reaching epidemic proportion (as it has already elsewhere in sub-Saharan Africa, such as Rwanda and the Congo). I was struck by the literal nature of the warnings about AIDS that I read plastered in the street, in shops and on the bulletin board in workers' libraries. Posters with words in eleven languages, posters with cautionary images, posters with instructions about condom use. But little attention was given to the trauma that the dying body evokes for the living. Of all nations in the world, South Africa is the one that is at present attempting to raise the questions of memories of the political past, of the victims and their identification and necessary reparations, of the trauma that marked and marks the body politic. But the public health officials in the 'new' South Africa do not quite understand that another trauma marks the South African memory of the past and its engagement with the future, and that is the ongoing presence of AIDS. Indeed, this issue is even more submerged in the 'new' South Africa than questions of gender, for the Western association of AIDS with homosexuality (in spite of the rampant presence of heterosexually transmitted HIV in sub-Saharan Africa) makes the topic truly taboo in South Africa. An anxiety about 'sexual deviance' seems deeply rooted in all the South African communities.

Some few visual artists there (unlike the public health officials) understand this well. Censorship and self-censorship of sexual material in high and mass art is rampant. Kendell Geers, one of the most original and provocative artists now living in South Africa, understands the relationship between censorship and danger.[6] In an exhibition in the summer of 1994 he had the viewer move into one of three gallery spaces through a room smeared from floor to ceiling with dried animal blood. The multiple meaning of blood – including that of AIDS – must be confronted. (Geers had organized South African artists in an exhibit of 'AIDS-art' entitled 'AIDS: The Exhibit' a few years earlier.) One might add that Geer's exhibit, when it was first installed, stank. It stank of blood – not human blood, but animal blood – but stank none the less. With time only the memory of the smell remained. The spur of the smell, the smell of decay, the smell that we all fear in our own bodies – so carefully washed and sprayed and perfumed – the smell of dying, remained to engage the viewer. Trapped in this windowless room, the smell and the sight of dried blood present in every fibre of my being, the world of AIDS evoking my repressed memories of the past and my anxieties about my own stability. This anxiety is lacking in the cool, distant, often comically clinical public health posters that one sees sporadically on the streets of Johannesburg.

And yet Geers's 1994 exhibit was equally problematic in its need to place the visceral aspect of AIDS in a historical context. In one of the other two venues for the exhibits, the famed Market Gallery, the work evoked the Shoah in a direct manner. The viewer entered into that gallery on a staircase above which was inscribed 'Arbeit macht Frei' ('Work liberates'), the motto that was part of the gate of Auschwitz. One was then confronted with an elaborate, brightly shining swirl of razor-wire, razor-wire that, according to Geers, symbolically evoked apartheid as well as the barbed wire of the death camps. Geers's easy parallel among the visual worlds of apartheid, AIDS and the Shoah discomforted me because it created a sense of universal victimization linked through a vocabulary of well-worn images. Apartheid and AIDS became yet two further 'holocausts', losing their historical particularity. Unlike the visceral effect of his 'blood room', these references were cerebral. In was clear that Geers, too, found the received imagery of the Shoah compelling, and yet, in employing it, he worked against his own project of making AIDS a unique moment in the complex post-Shoah, South African history of representing blood, dissolution and death. If Geers's room of blood was 'ugly' because of its physical association with dissolution and decay, the swirl of razor-wire was strangely and unpleasantly beautiful, its polished surface more reminiscent of a David Smith sculpture than the rusted, bloodstained strands of barbed wire at Dachau, Belsen or Auschwitz. Such meta-images exist separate from space and time as part of a construct of the distanced and controlled world of the 'aesthetic'. And they demean the experience of all those whose victim status is thus compared. Here too, the image becomes a means of controlling the anxiety about the transience of one's own positionality.

Images of health and illness seem to be interchangeable with those of beauty and ugliness in Western societies. Whether in the history of the nose or the world of official AIDS imagery, there is an easy parallel that Western cultures (including medical culture) have drawn. Thus even patients are so constructed by physicians so as to emphasize this association. 'Beautiful' patients (the young and the female) are held to be 'good' patients. They will obey the doctor's wishes and they will get better. 'Ugly' patients (the 'old') will transgress the doctor's will and they will inevitably die.[7] But, of course, all patients inevitably die, as do all doctors. It is this anxiety that is placed in abeyance when the visual stereotypes of appearance are used as absolute cues to the state of mind and body. In the historians' study of images of health and illness, the analysis of these cultural fantasies about the function of the visual world should be at the very centre. This book has, I hope, continued that analysis in new and different directions. This is not a conclusion.

References

1. How and Why do Historians of Medicine Use or Ignore Images

1 Frances Haskell, *History and Its Images: Art and the Interpretation of the Past* (New Haven, 1993); Michael Baxandall, *Patterns of Intention: On the Historical Explanation of Pictures* (New Haven, 1985); Irving Lavin, *Past-Present: Essays on Historicism in Art from Donatello to Picasso* (Berkeley, 1993); Peter Paret, *Art as History: Episodes in the Culture and Politics of Nineteenth-century Germany* (Princeton, 1988); Simon Schama, *The Embarrassment of Riches: An Interpretation of Dutch Culture in the Golden Age* (New York, 1987); Theodore K. Rabb, *The Struggle for Stability in Early Modern Europe* (New York, 1975).

2 Peter Gay, *Art and Act: On Causes in History – Manet, Gropius, Mondrian* (New York, 1976).

3 Arnaldo Momigliano, 'Ancient History and the Antiquarian', *Journal of the Warburg and Courtauld Institute*, III/IV (1950), pp. 285–315.

4 On this question see the papers collected in Robert I. Rotberg and Theodore K. Rabb, eds., *Art and History: Images and their Meaning* (Cambridge and New York, 1988).

5 Felix Marti-Ibañez, ed., *The Epic of Medicine* (New York, [1962]).

6 Maxime Laignel-Lavastine, *Histoire générale de la médecine, de la pharmacie, de l'art dentaire et de l'art vétérinaire; ornée de nombreuses illustrations*, 3 vols (Paris, 1936–49).

7 Arnaldo Cherubini, *I Medici Scrittori dal XV al XX secolo* (Rome, 1977), p. 293.

8 Nancy Duin and Jenny Sutcliffe, *A History of Medicine: From Prehistory to the Year 2020* (New York, 1992), p. 6.

9 Ann G. Carmichael and Richard M. Ratzan, eds., *Medicine: A Treasury of Art and Literature* (New York, 1991).

10 See, for example, George A. Bender, *Great Moments in Medicine: A Collection of the First Thirty Stories and Paintings in the Continuing Series 'A History of Medicine in Pictures'*, paintings by Robert A. Thom (Detroit, 1961); Albert S. Lyons and R. Joseph Petrucelli, *Medicine: An Illustrated History* (New York, 1978); Richard Toellner, ed., *Illustrierte Geschichte der Medizin*, 9 vols (Salzburg, 1980); Jean-Charles Sournia, *The Illustrated History of Medicine*, trans. Louise Davies, Graham Cross and Lilian Hall (London, 1992); Rick Smolan, *Medicine's Great Journey: One Hundred Years of Healing*, created by Rick Smolan and Phillip Moffitt; intro. by Robert Coles; text by Richard Flaste (Boston, 1992).

11 Abraham Aaron Roback and Thomas Kiernan, *Pictorial History of Psychology and Psychiatry* (New York, 1969).

12 Josephine A. Dolan, M. Louise Fitzpatrick and Eleanor Krohn Herrmann, *Nursing in Society: A Historical Perspective* (Philadelphia, 1983); M. Patricia Donahue, *Nursing, The Finest Art: An Illustrated History* (St Louis, 1985); Madeleine Masson, *A Pictorial History of Nursing* (London, 1985).

13 Art Newman, *The Illustrated Treasury of Medical Curiosa* (New York, 1988).

14 Lyons and Petrucelli, *op. cit.*, p. 8.

15 Jim Harter, *Images of Medicine* (New York, 1991), p. ix.

16 Helmut Vogt, *Der Arzt am Krankenbett: Eine Charakteristik in Bildern aus fünf Jahrhunderten* (Munich, 1984).

17 Joel-Peter Witkin, *Masterpieces of Medical Photography: Selections for the Burns Archive* (Pasadena, CA, 1987), p. [1].

18 Renata Taureck, *Die Bedeutung der Photographie für die medizinische Abbildung im 19. Jahrhundert* (Cologne: Forschungsstelle des Instituts für die Geschichte der Medizin, 1980).

19 Daniel M. Fox and Christopher Lawrence, *Photographing Medicine: Images and Power in Britain and America since 1840* (New York, 1988).

20 Harold I. Kaplan and Benjamin J. Sadock, *Comprehensive Textbook of Psychiatry*, 5th edn (Baltimore, 1989).

21 John L. Thornton and Carole Reeves, *Medical Book Illustration: A Short History* (Cambridge, 1983), p. 15.

22 Robert Herrlinger, *Geschichte der medizinischen Abbildung*, 2 vols (Munich, 1967–72).

23 André Hahn and Paule Dumaitre, *Histoire de la médecine et du livre médical* (Paris, 1962).

24 Ludwig Choulant, *Geschichte und Bibliographie der anatomischen Abbildung nach ihrer Beziehung auf anatomische Wissenschaft und bildende Kunst* (Leipzig, 1852).

25 Hans Schadewalt, Léon Binet, Charles Maillant and Ilza Veith, *Kunst und Medizin* (Cologne, 1967).

26 A small selection of such studies would be Carl Zigrosser, *Ars medica: A Collection of Medical Prints Presented to the Laboratories* [Philadelphia, 1959]; Loren Carey MacKinney, *Medical Illustrations in Medieval Manuscripts* (London, 1965); Ernst Berger, *Das Basler Arztrelief. Studien zum griechischen Grab- und Votivrelief um 500 v. Chr. und zur vorhippokratischen Medizin* (Basle, 1970); Veit Harold Bauer, *Das Antonius-Feuer in Kunst und Medizin* (Basle, 1973); Anton Seidenbusch, *Kunst und Medizin in Padua: Beruhrpunkte zwischen Heilkunde und bildender Kunst, dargestellt anhand von Beispielen aus Paduas Kirchen und der Scuola del Santo* (Pattensen, 1975); Heide Grape-Albers, *Spätantike Bilder aus der Welt des Arztes: medizinische Bilderhandschriften der Spätantike und ihre mittelalterliche Überlieferung* (Wiesbaden, 1977); Jorgen Schmidt-Voigt, *Russische Ikonenmalerei und Medizin* (Munich, 1980); *The Art of Healing: Medicine and Science in American Art*, exhibition catalogue by William H. Gerdts: Birmingham Museum of Art (Birmingham, AL, 1981); Wilhelm Theopold, *Votivmalerei und Medizin: Kulturgeschichte und Heilkunst im Spiegel der Votivmalerei* (Munich, 1981); Peter Murray Jones, *Medieval Medical Miniatures* (London, 1984); Kitti Jurina, *Vom Quacksalber zum Doctor Medicinae: die Heilkunde in der deutschen Graphik des 16, Jahrhunderts* (Cologne, 1985); *Ars medica, Art, Medicine, and the Human Condition: Prints, Drawings, and Photographs from the Collection of the Philadelphia Museum of Art*, exhibition catalogue by Diane R. Karp (Philadelphia, 1985).

27 See, for example, Friedrich von Zglinicki, *Die Uroskopie in der bildenden Kunst: eine kunst- und medizinhistorische Untersuchung über die Harnschau* (Darmstadt, 1982).

28 See, for example, Axel Hinrich Murken, *Joseph Beuys und die Medizin* (Munster, 1979), and *Herbert Boeckl, die Bilder und Zeichnungen zur Anatomie*, exhibition catalogue: Salzburger Landessammlungen Rupertinum; Kulturhaus der Stadt Graz (Salzburg, 1984).

29 On Eugen Holländer and his studies, see below. For more contemporary studies see Helmut Vogt, *Medizinische Karikaturen von 1800 bis zur Gegenwart* (Munich, 1960); *The Picture of Health: Images of Medicine and Pharmacy from the William H. Helfand Collection*, exhibition catalogue by William H. Helfand: Philadelphia

Museum of Art (Philadelphia, 1991), and William H. Helfand, *Medicine and Pharmacy in American Political Prints, 1765–1870* (Madison, WI: American Institute of the History of Pharmacy, 1978).

30 Charles Rosenberg, 'Framing Disease: Illness, Society and History', in his *Explaining Epidemics and Other Studies in the History of Medicine* (Cambridge, 1992), pp. 305–18. See also Rosenberg's edited volume with Janet Golden, *Framing Disease: Studies in Cultural History* (New Brunswick, NJ, 1992).

31 Sander L. Gilman, *The Face of Madness: Hugh W. Diamond and the Rise of Psychiatric Photography* (New York, 1976); *Seeing the Insane: A Cultural History of Psychiatric Illustration* (New York, 1982); *Disease and Representation: Images of Illness from Madness to AIDS* (Ithaca, NY, 1988).

32 George Didi-Huberman, *Invention de l'hystérie: Charcot et l'iconographie photographique de la Salpêtrière* (Paris, 1982); Elaine Showalter, *The Female Malady: Women, Madness, and English Culture, 1830–1980* (New York, 1985); Michael Fried, *Realism, Writing, Disfiguration: On Thomas Eakins and Stephen Crane* (Chicago, 1987); Ludmilla Jordanova, *Sexual Visions: Images of Gender in Science and Medicine between the Eighteenth and Twentieth Centuries* (Madison, WI, 1989); Barbara Maria Stafford, *Body Criticism: Imaging the Unseen in Enlightenment Art and Medicine* (Cambridge, MA, 1992).

33 Kathy Newman, 'Wounds and Wounding in the American Civil War: A Visual History', *The Yale Journal of Criticism*, VI (1993), pp. 63–86.

34 The most accessible edition is the English translation: Hans Prinzhorn, *Artistry of the Mentally Ill: A Contribution to the Psychology and Psychopathology of Configuration*, trans. Eric von Brockdorff (New York, 1972).

35 One of the first monographs on the topic dedicated to the work of a single artist has recently been made available in English: Walter Morgenthaler, *Madness and Art: The Life and Works of Adolf Wölfli*, trans. Aaron H. Esman (Lincoln, NB, 1992).

36 See, for example, Maria Meurer-Keldenich, *Medizinische Literatur zur Bildnerei von Geisteskranken* (Cologne: Forschungsstelle des Instituts fur Geschichte der Medizin der Universität zu Köln, 1979); *The Prinzhorn Collection: Selected Work from the Prinzhorn Collection of the Art of the Mentally Ill*, exhibition catalogue by Stephen Prokopoff: Krannert Art Museum, University of Illinois; Lowe Art Museum, Miami; David and Alfred Smart Gallery, Chicago; Herbert F. Johnson Museum of Art, Ithaca, NY (Champaign, IL, 1984); John M. MacGregor, *The Discovery of the Art of the Insane* (Princeton, NJ, 1989).

37 *Parallel Visions: Modern Artists and Outsider Art*, exhibition catalogue by Maurice Tuchman and Carol S. Eliel: Los Angeles County Museum of Art; Museo Nacional, Reina Sofia, Madrid; Kunsthalle Basel; Setegaya Art Museum, Tokyo (Princeton, NJ, 1992).

38 Louis Arnorsson Sass, *Madness and Modernism: Insanity in the Light of Modern Art, Literature, and Thought* (New York, 1992).

39 An exception is to be found in Sournia, *op. cit.*, p. 526.

40 Haskell, *op. cit.*, p. 331ff.

41 Georges Canguilhem, *The Normal and the Pathological*, trans. Carolyn R. Fawcett (Boston, 1989).

42 See Haskell, *op. cit.*, p. 346ff.

43 On Charcot's biography see A. R. G. Owen, *Hysteria, Hypnosis and Healing: The Work of J.-M. Charcot* (London, 1971), and Georges Guillain, *J.-M. Charcot, 1825–1893: His Life – His Work* (New York, 1959).

44 Elizabeth Cartwright, 'Physiological Modernism: Cinematography as a Medical Research Technology', dissertation, Yale, 1991.

45 Toby Gelfand, ' "Mon Cher Docteur Freud": Charcot's Unpublished Correspondence to Freud, 1888–1893', *Bulletin of the History of Medicine*, LXII (1988), pp. 563–88, here, p. 571.

46 See Jean-Martin Charcot and Paul Richer, *Les démoniaques dans l'art* (Paris, 1887) and their *Les difformes et les malades dans l'art* (Paris, 1889) as well as numerous articles on the relationship between the artistic representations of madness and psychiatric nosologies in Charcot's house journal *Nouvelle iconographie de la Salpêtrière: clinique des maladies du système nerveux* (Paris, 1888–1918).

47 This is true in his 'medical' writing, such as Paul Richer, *Études cliniques sur la grande hystérie ou hystéro-épilepsie*, 2nd revd edn (Paris, 1885), as well as in his 'art history', *L'art et la médecine* (Paris, 1900).

48 J. Aguayo, 'Charcot and Freud: Some Implications of Late Nineteenth-century French Psychiatry and Politics for the Origins of Psychoanalysis', *Psychoanalysis and Contemporary Thought*, IX (1986), pp. 223–60.

49 Sigmund Freud, *The Standard Edition of the Complete Psychological Works*, ed. and trans. J. Strachey, A. Freud, A. Strachey and A. Tyson, 24 vols (London, 1955–74), I, p. 17.

50 The result is quite striking, even within France. See Martin Jay, *Downcast Eyes: The Denigration of Vision in Twentieth-century French Thought* (Berkeley, CA, 1993).

51 See Dirk Friedrich Rodekirchen, *Karl Sudhoff (1853–1938) und die Anfänge der Medizin-Geschichte in Deutschland*, dissertation, Cologne, 1992.

52 See, for example, Karl Sudhoff, *Mal Franzoso in Italien in der ersten Hälfte des 15. Jahrhunderts; ein Blatt aus der Geschichte der Syphilis* (Giessen, 1912); ed., *Graphische und typographische Erstlinge der Syphilis-Literatur aus den Jahren 1495 und 1496* (Munich, 1912); Sudhoff and Moriz Hall, eds, *Des Andreas Vesalius sechs anatomische Tafeln vom Jahre 1538 in Lichtdruck, neu herausgegeben und der 86. Versammlung Deutscher Naturforscher und Aerzte zur Feier der 400. Wiederkehr des Jahres seiner Geburt* (Leipzig, 1920); ed., *Zehn Syphilis-Drucke aus den Jahren 1495–1498* (Milan, 1924), English trans. as *The Earliest Printed Literature on Syphilis being Ten Tractates from the Years 1495–1498. In complete facsimile with an introduction and other accessory material by Karl Sudhoff; adapted by Charles Singer* (Florence, 1925); Sudhoff and Max Geisberg, eds, *Die anatomischen Tafeln des Jost de Negker 1539, mit 6 Tafeln und 2 Abbildungen im Text* (Munich, 1928).

53 Karl Sudhoff, 'Photographie oder Zeichnung?', *Wochenschrift für klassische Philologie* XXVIII (1911), col. 279; 'Medizin und Kunst. Ein Wort der Einführung und Weihe', *Katalog zur Ausstellung der Geschichte der Medizin in Kunst und Kunstwerk. Zur Eröffnung des Kaiserin-Friedrich-Hauses in Berlin 1906* (Stuttgart, 1906), pp. 21–6.

54 Karl Sudhoff, 'Abermals eine neue Handschrift der anatomischen Fünfbilderserie', *Archiv für Geschichte der Medizin*, III (1909), pp. 353–68.

55 Theodor Puschmann, 'Die Bedeutung der Geschichte für die Medicin und die Naturwissenschaften,' *Deutsche medizinische Wochenschrift*, XV (1889), pp. 817–20.

56 Karl Sudhoff, 'Theodor Puschmann und die Aufgaben der Geschichte der Medizin. Eine akademische Antrittsvorlesung', *Müncher medizinische Wochenschrift*, LIII (1906), p. 270.

57 Henry Ernest Sigerist, *Civilization and Disease* (Ithaca, NY, 1943).

58 Ernst Schwalbe, *Vorlesungen über Geschichte der Medizin*, 3rd edn (Jena, 1920).

59 Theodor Meyer-Steineg and Karl Sudhoff, *Geschichte der Medizin im Überblick mit Abbildungen* (Jena, 1921).

60 Theodor Meyer-Steineg and Karl Sudhoff, *Illustrierte Geschichte der Medizin*. 5th edn, ed. Robert Herrlinger and Fridolf Kudlien (Stuttgart, 1965).

61 Theodor Meyer-Steineg, *Chirurgische Instrumente des Altertums: ein Beitrag zur antiken Akiurgie* (Jena, 1912), and *Darstellungen normaler und krankhaft veränderter Körperteile an antiken Weihgaben* (Jena, 1912).

62 Theodor Meyer-Steineg, 'Geschichte der Medizin als Lehrgegenstand', *Berliner klinische Wochenschrift*, LVII (1920), p. 158.

63 See Fielding H. Garrison, *John Shaw Billings: A Memoir* (New York, 1915), pp. 234–5, and John S. Haller, Jr, 'The Artful Science: Medicine's Self-Image in the 1890s', *Clio Medica*, XIX (1984), pp. 231–50.

64 Hermann Peters, *Der Arzt und die Heilkunst in alten Zeiten* (Leipzig, 1900).

65 Eugen Holländer, *Die Medizin in der klassischen Malerei* (Stuttgart, 1903); *Die Karikatur und Satire in der Medizin: Mediko-kunsthistorische Studie. Mit 10 farbigen Tafeln und 223 Abbildungen im Text* (Stuttgart, 1905); *Plastik und Medizin* (Stuttgart, 1912); *Die Medizin in der klassichen Malerei*, 2nd edn (Stuttgart, 1913); *Die Karikatur und Satire in der Medizin. Mediko-kunsthistorische Studie*, 2nd edn, *Mit 11 farbigen Tafeln und 251 Abbildungen im Text.* (Stuttgart, 1921); *Wunder, Wundergeburt und Wundergestalt in einblattdrucken des fünfzehnten bis achtzehnten Jahrhunderts* (Stuttgart, 1921); *Die Medizin in der klassischen Malerei. Mit 272 in den Text gedruckten Abbildungen*, 3rd edn (Stuttgart, 1923); *Äskulap und Venus: eine Kultur- und Sittengeschichte im Spiegel des Arztes* (Berlin, 1928).

66 Karl Sudhoff, 'Plastik und Medizin. Eine glossierende Besprechung des gleichnamigen Werkes Eugen Holländers', *Zeitschrift für Balneologie*, V (1912–13), pp. 461–7. What Sudhoff undertakes in this review is to compliment Holländer on his coverage and then provide page upon page of variant readings of the material he brings from ancient Greek medical iconography.

67 See Holländer's statement in *Plastik und Medizin, op. cit.*, p. 2, and *Die Karikatur und Satire in der Medizin, op. cit.*, p. 3.

68 Michel Foucault, *The Foucault Reader*, ed. Paul Rabinow (New York, 1984), p. 199.

2. Again Madness as a Test Case

1 See Joseph Guislain, *Traité sur l'aliénation mentale et sur les hospices des aliénés* (Amsterdam, 1826), as well as his *Klinische Vorträge über Geistes-Krankheiten*, trans. Heinrich Laehr (Berlin, 1854).

2 I am grateful for discussions with Bruno-Nassim Aboudar of Paris concerning his dissertation on the image of the insane before the invention of photography.

3 Richard T. Gray, 'Lavater's Physiognomical "Surface Hermeneutics" and the Ideological (Con-)Text of Bourgeois Modernism', *Lessing Yearbook*, XXIII (1991), pp. 127–48, here p. 137.

4 See August Krauss, 'Der Sinn im Wahnsinn', *Allgemeine Zeitschrift für Psychiatrie*, XVII (1859), pp. 10–35, as well as his *Die Psychologie des Verbrechens. Ein Beitrag zur Erfahrungsseelenkunde* (Tübingen, 1884).

5 William Bynum and Roy Porter, eds, *Medicine and the Five Senses* (Cambridge, 1993).

6 See *George Bellows: The Artist and his Lithographs, 1916–1924*, exhibition catalogue by Jane Myers and Linda Ayres: Amon Carter Museum (Fort Worth, 1988); Lauris Mason, *The Lithographs of George Bellows: A Catalogue Raisonné* (San Francisco, 1992); Marianne Doezema, *George Bellows and Urban America* (New Haven, 1992).

7 Isaac Newton Kerlin, *The Mind Unveiled: or, a Brief History of Twenty-two Imbecile Children* (Philadelphia, 1858).

8 On this image see G. M. Wilson, 'Early Photography, Goitre, and James Inglis', *British Medical Journal* (14 April 1973), pp. 104–5; F. Merke, *History and Iconography of Endemic Goitre and Cretinism* (Boston, 1984); A. Giampalmo and E. Fulcheri, 'An Investigation of Endemic Goitre during the Centuries in Sacral Figurative Arts', *Zentralblatt für allgemeine Pathologie*, LXI (1988), pp. 297–307; B. S. Hetzel, 'The History of Goitre and Cretinism', in his *The Story of Iodine Deficiency: The Challenge of Prevention* (Oxford, 1989), pp. 3–20.

9 Freud, *op. cit.*, IX, p. 72.

3. *The Ugly and the Beautiful*

1 Jules Hércourt, *The Social Diseases: Tuberculosis, Syphilis, Alcoholism, Sterility*, trans. with a final chapter by Bernard Miall (London, 1920), pp. 244–5.

2 An excellent overview of this question from the standpoint of the earlier theories of medical physiognomy is Barbara M. Stafford, John La Puma, and David L. Schiedermayer, 'One Face of Beauty, One Picture of Health: The Hidden Aesthetic of Medical Practice', *Journal of Medicine and Philosophy*, XIV (1989), pp. 213–30.

3 W. H. S. Jones, ed. and trans., *Hippocrates*, 6 vols (Cambridge, 1959), II, p. 311.

4 George A. Aitken, ed., *The Tatler*, 4 vols (London, 1899), IV, p. 162.

5 Cited by D. J. Enright, ed., *Ill at Ease: Writers on Ailments Real and Imagined* (London, 1989), p. 3.

6 Wilhelm Weischedel, ed., *Immanuel Kant, Werke*, 10 vols (Darmstadt, 1975), VIII, pp. 283–7.

7 Karl Rosenkranz, *Ästhetik des Häßlichen* (1853; Leipzig, 1990), pp. 5–8.

8 Georges Canguilhem, *The Normal and the Pathological*, trans. Carolyn R. Fawcett (Boston, 1989).

9 On the general problem of the Black as the marker for racial ugliness in the eighteenth and nineteenth centuries see my *On Blackness without Blacks: Essays on the Image of the Black in Germany*, Yale Afro-American Studies (Boston, 1982), pp. 19–35.

10 Friedrich Nietzsche, *The Genealogy of Morals*, trans. Francis Golffing (New York, 1956), pp. 167–8.

11 Anna Fischer-Duckelmann, *Die Frau als Hausärtzin: Ein ärztliches Nachschlagebuch der Gesundheitspflege und Heilkunde in der Familie* (1901; Stuttgart, 1905).

12 See, for example, Thomas Ewell, *The Ladies' Medical Companion: Containing, In A Series Of Letters, An Account Of The Latest Improvements And Most Successful Means Of Preserving Their Beauty And Health; Of Relieving The Diseases Peculiar To The Sex, And An Explanation Of The Offices They Should Perform To Each Other At Births. With Engraved Figures Explanatory. Also, The Best Means Of Nursing, Preventing And Curing The Diseases Of Children . . .* (Philadelphia, 1818); Alexander Walker, *Intermarriage: Or, The Mode In Which, And The Causes Why, Beauty, Health And Intellect, Result From Certain Unions, And Deformity, Disease And Insanity, From Others . . .* (New York, 1839); Jean Dubois, MD, *The Secret Habits Of The Female Sex: Letters Addressed To A Mother On The Evils Of Solitude, And Its Seductive Temptations To Young Girls, The Premature Victims Of A Pernicious Passion, With All Its Frightful Consequences; Deformity Of Mind And Body, Destruction Of Beauty, And Entailing Disease And Death: But From Which, By Attention To The Timely Warning Here Given, The Devotee May Be Saved, And Become An Ornament To Society, A Virtuous Wife And A Refulgent Mother: This Work Should Be Read By All Classes; While It Forcibly Describes The Misery Attendant Upon Solitude, It Prescribes A Medical Treatment And Regimen Which Has Never Failed Of Success*, from the French of Jean Dubois, MD (Philadelphia: sold by the booksellers generally [186–?]); Benjamin Franklin Scholl, *Library Of Health: Complete Guide To Prevention And Cure Of Disease, Containing Practical Information On Anatomy, Physiology and Preventive Medicine; Curative Medicine, First Aid Measures, Diagnosis, Nursing, Sexology, Simple Home Remedies, Care Of The Teeth, Occupational Diseases, Garden Plant Remedies, Alcohol And Narcotics, Treatment By Fifteen Schools Of Medicine, Beauty Culture, Physical Culture, The Science Of Breathing And The Dictionary Of Drugs. Twenty Books – One Volume* (Philadelphia, [c. 1916]).

13 Ernst Brücke, *Schönheit und Fehler der menschlichen Gestalt* (Vienna, 1891), pp. 141–4.

14 See my *The Jew's Body* (New York, 1992), pp. 38–59.

15 Immanuel Kant, *Observations of the Feeling of the Beautiful and Sublime*, trans. John T. Goldthwait (Berkeley, 1960), p. 87.

16 Barbara Freeman, 'The Rise of the Sublime: Sacrifice and Misogyny in Eighteenth-century Aesthetics', *Yale Journal of Criticism*, IV (1992), pp. 81–99.

17 All references are to Anatole Leroy-Beaulieu, *Israel Among the Nations: A Study of the Jews and Antisemitism*, trans. Frances Hellman (New York, 1895), here p. 247. This was first published as Anatole Leroy-Beaulieu (i.e. Henry Jean Baptiste Anatole), *(Les) juifs et l'antisémitisme: Israël chez les nations* (Paris, 1893). This went through at least seven printings in 1893 alone! Of his other works, see *La Révolution et le libéralisme; essais de critique et d'histoire* (Paris, 1890) and his pamphlet *Les immigrants juifs et le judaïsme aux États-Unis* (Paris, 1905). On his work see the following, which, though of less interest for our topic, has much information on the image of the East: Martha Helms Cooley, 'Nineteenth-century French Historical Research on Russia: Louis Leger, Alfred Rambaud, Anatole Leroy-Beaulieu', dissertation, Indiana, 1971.

18 Sander L, Gilman, *Difference and Pathology: Stereotypes of Sexuality, Race, and Madness* (Ithaca, NY, 1985), pp. 76–109.

19 Richard Burke, *A Historical Chronology of Tuberculosis* (Springfield, 1938), p. 17.

20 Max Neuberger, 'Zur Geschichte der Konstitutionslehre', *Zeitschrift für angewandte Anatomie und Konstitutionslehre*, I (1914), pp. 4–10.

21 Christoph Wilhelm Hufeland, *Enchiridion medicum: or The Practice of Medicine*, trans. Caspar Bruchhausen (1836; New York, 1844), pp. 285, 288.

22 Albert Reibmayr, *Die Ehe Tuberkuloser und Ihre Folgen* (Leipzig/Vienna, 1894).

23 F. Köhler, 'Die psychische Einwirkung', *Beiträge zur Klinik der Tuberkulose*, XXII (1912), supplement 3, pp. 2–8, here p. 4.

24 Robert Jütte, 'Stigma-Symbole: Kleidung als identitätsstiftendes Merkmal bei spätmittelalterlichen und frührneuzeitlichen Randgruppen (Juden, Dirnen, Aussätzige, Bettler),' *Saeculum*, XLIV (1993), pp. 65–89.

25 George L. Mosse, *Nationalism and Sexuality: Middle-class Morality and Sexual Norms in Modern Europe* (New York, 1985), pp. 133–52.

4. *The Phantom of the Opéra's Nose*

1 All quotations are from Gaston Leroux, *The Phantom of the Opéra*, intro. by Max Byrd (New York, 1987), here p. 9.

2 Ashley Montagu, *The Elephant Man: A Study in Human Dignity* (New York, 1971); Michael Howell, *The True History of the Elephant Man* (London, 1980); Peter W. Graham, *Articulating the Elephant Man: Joseph Merrick and his Interpreters* (Baltimore, 1992).

3 Nikolai Gogol, *Diary of a Madman and Other Stories*, trans. Ronald Wilks (New York, 1972), p. 56.

4 Edgar Allan Poe, *Poetry and Tales* (New York, 1984), p. 217.

5 Walter de la Mare, *Broomsticks and Other Tales* (London, 1925), pp. 175–226.

6 William Saroyan, *The Human Comedy* (New York, 1943), p. 63.

7 See Gaspare Tagliacozzi, *La Chirurgia Plastica per Innesto*, trans. and ed. Werner Vallieri (Bologna, 1964), and the standard monograph on him by Martha Teach Gnudi and Jerome Pierce Webster, *The Life and Times of Gaspare Tagliacozzi, Surgeon of Bologna 1545–1599* (New York, 1950).

8 See, for example, Blair O. Rogers, 'A Brief History of Cosmetic Surgery', *Surgical Clinics of North America*, LI (1971), pp. 265–88, as well as his 'A Chronological History of Cosmetic Surgery', *Bulletin of the New York Academy of Medicine*, XLVII (1971), pp. 265–302.

9 John Bulwer, *Anthropometamorphosis: Man Transform'd: OR, The Artificiall Changling Historically Presented* (London, 1653), p. C *verso*.

10 Margaret Pelling, 'Appearance and Reality: Barber-Surgeons, the Body and Disease', in A. L. Beier and Roger Finlay, eds, *London 1500–1700: The Making of the Metropolis* (London, 1986), pp. 82–112, here p. 94.

11 Donald F. Bond, ed., The *Tatler* (Oxford, 1987), III, pp. 317–22.

12 Richard Selzer, 'The Sympathetic Nose', in his *Rituals of Surgery* (New York, 1974), pp. 37–49.

13 Dr. Klein, 'Über Rhinoplastick', *Heidelberger Klinische Annalen*, II (1826), pp. 103–11.

14 The 'saddle-nose' is also the most visible mark of the physiognomy of the Black in the eighteenth and nineteenth centuries; it becomes the shorthand for representing the inferiority of the character and intelligence of the African. For a detailed discussion of this see my *On Blackness without Blacks: Essays on the Image of the Black in Germany*. Yale Afro-American Studies (Boston, 1982), pp. 19–34.

15 J. S. Carey, 'Kant and the Cosmetic Surgeon', *Journal of the Florida Medical Association*, LXXVI (1989), pp. 637–43.

16 Wilhelm Weygandt, *Atlas und Grundriss der Psychiatrie* (Munich, 1902).

17 John O. Roe, 'The Deformity Termed "Pug Nose" And its Correction, by a Simple Operation' (1887), reprinted in Frank McDowell, ed., *The Source Book of Plastic Surgery* (Baltimore, 1977), pp. 114–9, here 114.

18 Mary Cowling, *The Artist as Anthropologist: The Representation of Type and Character in Victorian Art* (Cambridge, 1989), pp. 125–29.

19 Paolo Mantegazza, *Physiognomy and Expression* (London, 1904), p. 45.

20 Peter Camper, *Der natüraliche Unterschied der Gesichtszüge in Menschen verschiedener Gegenden und verschiedenen Alters*, trans. S. Th. Sömmering (Berlin, 1792).

21 Sander L. Gilman, *The Jew's Body* (New York, 1991).

22 'Docteur Celticus', *Les 19 Tares corporelles visibles pour reconnaître un juif* (Paris, 1903).

23 Paul Narvig, *Jacques Joseph: Surgical Sculptor* (Philadelphia, 1982), pp. 23–4.

24 Stephan Mencke, *Zur Geschichte der Orthopädie* (Munich, 1930), pp. 68–80.

25 Bruno Valentin, *Geschichte der Orthopädie* (Stuttgart, 1961), pp. 101–2.

26 Mario González-Ulloa, ed., *The Creation of Aesthetic Plastic Surgery* (New York, 1985), pp. 87–114.

27 Jacques Joseph, 'Über die operative Verkleinerung einer Nase (Rhinomiosis)', *Berliner klinische Wochenschrift*, XL (1898), pp. 882–85; trans. in Jacques Joseph, 'Operative Reduction of the Size of a Nose (Rhinomiosis)', trans. Gustave Aufricht, *Plastic and Reconstructive Surgery*, XLVI (1970), pp. 178–81; reproduced in Frank McDowell, ed., *The Source Book of Plastic Surgery, op. cit.*, pp. 164–7.

28 Used to illustrate Jacques Joseph, *Nasenplastik und sonstige Gesichtsplastik, nebst einem Anhang über Mammaplastik und einige weitere Operationen aus dem Gebiete der äusseren Körperplastik: Ein Atlas und ein Lehrbuch* (Leipzig, 1931).

29 Paul Schilder, *The Image and Appearance of the Human Body: Studies in the Constructive Energies of the Psyche* (New York, 1950).

30 Georg Mannheimer, *Lieder eines Juden* (Prague, 1937), p. 31.

31 V. D. Musset-Pathay, ed., *Jean-Jacques Rousseau, Oeuvres completes*, 4 vols (Paris, 1823), III, p. 20.

32 Alfred Berndorfer, 'Aesthetic Surgery as Organopsychic Therapy', *Aesthetic and Plastic Surgery*, III (1979), pp. 143–6, here p. 143.

5. *Mark Twain and Hysteria in the Holy Land*

1 In William Osler, *Men and Books*, ed. Earl F. Nation (Pasadena, CA, 1959), p. 56.
2 Mark Twain, *Concerning the Jews*, (Philadelphia, 1985). This edition has a good historical introduction, and all quotations are from this edition. See also Carl Dolmetsch, *'Our Famous Guest': Mark Twain in Vienna* (Athens, GA, 1992), as well as his 'Mark Twain and the Viennese Anti-Semites: New Light on "Concerning the Jews"', *Mark Twain Journal*, XIII (1985), pp. 10–17; Guido Fink, 'Al di qua della paroia: Gli ebrei di Henry James e di Mark Twain', in Guido Fink and Gabriella Morisco, eds, *Il recupero de testo: Aspetti della letteratura ebraico-americana* (Bologna, 1988), pp. 29–50. The general background in Twain's work can be judged based on the extracts in Janet Smith, ed., *Mark Twain on the Damned Human Race* (New York, 1962), and Maxwell Geismar, ed., *Mark Twain and the Three R's: Race, Religion, Revolution* (Indianapolis, 1973). The best overall discussion of Mark Twain's attitude toward the Jews is still to be found in Philip S. Foner, *Mark Twain, Social Critic* (New York, 1958), pp. 288–307, which documents in great detail the critical reception of this piece, including its use in the anti-Semitic propaganda of the early twentieth century. On the overall question of the image of the Jew in nineteenth-century American culture see Louis Harap, *The Image of the Jew in American Literature from Early Republic to Mass Immigration* (Philadelphia, 1974).
3 Marion A. Richmond, 'The Lost Source in Freud's "Comment on Anti-Semitism": Mark Twain', *Journal of the American Psychoanalytic Association*, XXVIII (1980), pp. 563–74.
4 Cited by Foner, *op. cit.*, p. 300.
5 All references are to the following edition: Mark Twain, *The Innocents Abroad/Roughing It* (New York, 1984). On the historical background for this volume see Dewey Ganzel, *Mark Twain Abroad: The Cruise of the 'Quaker City'* (Chicago, 1968), and Franklin Dickerson Walker, *Irreverent Pilgrims: Melville, Browne, and Mark Twain in the Holy Land* (Seattle, 1974).
6 See L. Belloni, 'Anatomica plastica: The Bologna Wax Models', *CIBA Symposium*, VIII (1960), pp. 84–7; François Cagnetta, 'La vie et l'œuvre de Gaetano Giulio Zummo', *Cereoplastica nella scienza e nell'arte series: Atti del I congresso internazionale. Biblioteca della Revista di storia delle scienze mediche e naturali*, XX (1977), pp. 489–501. On the religious background to this tradition see the following two catalogues and their general historical introductions: Benedetto Lanza *et al.*, *La cere anatomiche della Specola* (Florence, 1979), on the Florentine collection, and, on the Viennese collection, Konrad Allmer and Marlene Jantsch, eds, *Katalog der josephinischen Sammlung anatomischer und geburtshilflicher Wachspräparate im Institut für Geschichte der Medizin an der Universität Wien* (Graz-Cologne, 1965).
7 Henry Wadsworth Longfellow, *Outre Mer: A Pilgrimage beyond the Sea* (London, 1853), pp. 224–5.
8 Nathaniel Hawthorne, *Passages from the French and Italian Note-Books* (Boston and New York, 1871), p. 380.
9 One must note that such a specific use of death and decay is quite different from Twain's metaphoric use of death. See Stephen Cooper, 'Good Rotten Material for a Burial': The Overdetermined Death of Romance in *Life on the Mississippi*', *Literature and Psychology*, XXXVI (1990), pp. 78–9.
10 Patrice Boudelais and Andre Dodin, *Visages du choléra* (Paris, 1987).
11 *Mark Twain's Notebooks and Journals: Volume I (1855–1873)*, ed. Frederick Anderson, Michael B. Frank and Kenneth M. Sanderson (Berkeley, 1975), I, p. 438.
12 On Twain's theology see Susan K. Harris, *Mark Twain's Escape from Time: A Study of Patterns and Images* (Columbia, MO, 1982).

13 Quoted by Ganzel, *op. cit.*, p. 222.

14 Quoted by Harap, *op. cit.*, p. 349.

15 *The Autobiography of Mark Twain*, ed. Charles Neider (New York, 1975), p. 3.

16 See the discussion in Foner, *op. cit.*, pp. 288–9.

17 Friedrich Ratzel, *The History of Mankind*, trans. A. J. Butler, 3 vols (London, 1896), III, p. 183. The German edition appeared between 1885 and 1888. For a more detailed discussion see my *Jewish Self-Hatred: Anti-Semitism and the Hidden Language of the Jews* (Baltimore, 1986), pp. 216–7.

18 Richard Andree, *Zur Volkskunde der Juden* (Leipzig, 1881), pp. 24–5; trans. from Maurice Fishberg, 'Material for the Physical Anthropology of the Eastern European Jew', *Memoirs of the American Anthropological Association*, I (1905–7), pp. 6–7.

19 Johannes Buxtorf, *Synagoga Judaica* . . . (Basle, 1643), pp. 620–22.

20 Johann Jakob Schudt, *Jüdische Merkwürdigkeiten* (Frankfurt am Main, 1714–18), II, p. 369. On the later ideological life of this debate see Wolfgang Fritz Haug, *Die Faschisierung des bürgerlichen Subjekts: Die Ideologie der gesunden Normalität und die Ausrottungspolitiken im deutschen Faschismus* (West Berlin, 1986).

21 Johann Pezzl, *Skizze von Wien: Ein Kultur- und Sittenbild aus der josephinsichen Zeit*, ed. Gustav Gugitz and Anton Schlossar (Graz, 1923), pp. 107–8.

22 On the meaning of this disease in the medical literature of the period see the following dissertations on the topic: Michael Scheiba, *Dissertatio inauguralis medica, sistens quaedam plicae pathologica: Germ. Juden-Zopff, Polon, Koltun: quam . . . in Academia Albertina pro gradu doctoris . . . subjiciet defensurus Michael Scheiba* . . . (Regiomonti [1739]) and Hieronymus Ludolf, *Dissertatio inauguralis medica de plica, vom Juden-Zopff* . . . (Erfordiae [1724]).

23 Madison Marsh, 'Jews and Christians', *The Medical and Surgical Reporter* [Philadelphia], XXX (1874), pp. 343–4, here p. 343.

24 Marsh, *op. cit.*, p. 343.

25 See the debate following the presentation of Joseph Jacobs, 'On the Racial Characteristics of Modern Jews', *The Journal of the Anthropological Institute*, XVI (1886), pp. 23–63, here pp. 56 and 61.

26 Marsh, *op. cit.*, p. 344.

27 Ibid.

28 Joseph Krauskopf, *Sanitary Science: A Sunday Lecture* (Philadelphia, 1889), p. 7.

29 Ephraim M. Epstein, 'Have the Jews any Immunity from Certain Diseases?', *The Medical and Surgical Reporter* [Philadelphia], XXX, (1874), pp. 343–4, here p. 343.

30 Epstein, *op. cit.*, p. 341.

31 Ibid.

32 Carl Claus, *Grundzüge der Zoologie zum Gebrauche an Universitäten und höheren Lehranstalten sowie zum Selbststudium*, 2 vols (Marburg, 1872), II, p. 123.

33 Marsh, 'Have the Jews any Immunity from Certain Diseases?', pp. 132–4.

34 On the history of the concept see Sander L. Gilman and Steven T. Katz, eds, *Anti-Semitism in Times of Crisis* (New York, 1991), p. 29.

35 Peter Charles Remondino, *History of Circumcision from the Earliest Times to the Present. Moral and Physical Reasons for its Performance, with a History of Eunuchism, Hermaphroditism, etc., and of the Different Operations Practiced upon the Prepuce* (Philadelphia, 1891), p. 186. Remondino's book was only published in 1892, but he notes in his introduction that it had been written decades earlier.

36 Stuart Creighton Miller, *'Benevolent Assimilation': The American Conquest of the Philippines, 1899–1903* (New Haven, 1982), p. 75.

37 Sander L. Gilman, 'On the Nexus of Madness and Blackness', in my *Difference and Pathology: Stereotypes of Sexuality, Race, and Madness* (Ithaca, NY, 1985), pp. 131–49.

38 See George Frederickson, *The Black Image in the White Mind: The Debate about Afro-American Character and Destiny (1817–1914)* (New York, 1971).
39 Cited by Foner, *op. cit.*, p. 290.
40 See Eugene Levy, 'Is the Jew a White Man?: Press Reaction to the Leo Frank Case, 1913–1915', *Phylon*, XXXV (1974), pp. 212–22.
41 Clara Clemens, *My Father, Mark Twain* (New York, 1931), pp. 203–4.
42 Dolmetsch, *op. cit.*, p. 14.
43 Sander L. Gilman, 'The Jewish Genius', in my *The Jew's Body* (New York, 1991), pp. 128–49.

6. *The Beautiful Body and AIDS*

1 Simon Whatney, *Policing Desire: Pornography, Aids and the Media* (Minneapolis, 1987), p. 9.
2 See, for example, Diane M. Calhoun-French, 'On a Soapbox: All My Children and AIDS Education', in Diane Raymond, ed., *Sexual Politics and Popular Culture* (Bowling Green, 1990), pp. 112–8; Allison Fraiberg and David Porush, 'Of AIDS, Cyborgs, and Other Indiscretions: Resurfacing the Body in the Postmodern', *Postmodern Culture: An Electronic Journal of Interdisciplinary Criticism*, I (1991); 48 paragraphs; Rodney Buxton, 'After It Happened . . . : The Battle to Present AIDS in Television Drama', *The Velvet Light Trap*, XXVII (1991), pp. 37–48; Susan Sontag, *AIDS and its Metaphors* (New York, 1989); Lee Edelman, 'Seeing Things: Representation, the Scene of Surveillance, and the Spectacle of Gay Male Sex', in Diane Fuss, ed., *Inside/Out: Lesbian Theories, Gay Theories* (New York, 1991), pp. 93–118; George L. Dillon, *et al.*, 'Resisting the Public Discourse of AIDS', *Textual Practice*, III (1989), pp. 388–96.
3 Elizabeth Fee and Daniel Fox, 'The Contemporary Historiography of AIDS', *Journal of Social History*, XXIII (1989), pp. 303–14; Mirko Grmek, *History of AIDS: Emergence and Origin of a Modern Pandemic*, trans. Russell C. Maulitz and Jacalyn Duffin (Princeton, 1990).
4 Lucinda H. Keister, 'The Poster Collection at the National Library of Medicine', *Caduceus*, VI (1990), pp. 38–42.
5 William H. Helfand, 'Art in the Service of Public Health: The Illustrated Poster', *Caduceus*, VI (1990), pp. 1–37.
6 James Miller, ed., *Fluid Exchanges: Artists and Critics in the AIDS Crisis* (Buffalo, 1992); Allan Klusacek and Ken Morrison, eds, *A Leap in the Dark: AIDS, Art and Contemporary Cultures* (Montreal, 1992).
7 Frank Wagner, *AIDS – Eine Kunstausstellung Über Leben und Sterben* (Berlin, 1988). See also Robert Atkins, 'In Grief And Anger: Photographing People With AIDS', *Aperture*, CXIV (1989), pp. 70–2, and the recent exhibition *Gegendarstellung: Ethik und Ästhetik im Zeitalter von Aids*, Kunst Verein Hamburg; Kunstmuseum Luzern (Cologne, 1992).
8 Thomas Yingling, 'AIDS in America: Postmodern Governance, Identity, and Experience', in Diane Fuss, ed., *Inside/Out, op. cit.*, pp. 292–310, here p. 301.
9 Mario Wirz, *Es ist spät, ich kann nicht atmen: Ein nächtlicher Bericht* (Berlin, 1992), p. 62.
10 George Whitmore, 'Someone Was Here', *The New York Times Magazine* (31 January 1988), p. 16.
11 Compare the literary presentations in M. Elizabeth Osborn, ed., *The Way We Live Now: American Plays and the AIDS Crisis* (New York: Theatre Communications Group, 1990), and John Preston, ed., *Personal Dispatches: Writers Confront AIDS* (New York, 1989).
12 See J. Church, 'No, SPEW you!', *Documents*, I (1992), pp. 110–16, as well as the following texts by Cindy Patton, *Inventing AIDS* (New York, 1990); 'Safe Sex and

the Pornographic Vernacular', in Bad Object-Choices, ed., *How Do I Look?* (Seattle, 1991), pp. 31–64; *Sex and Germs: The Politics of* AIDS (Boston, 1985).

13 Douglas Crimp with Adam Rolston, AIDS *Demo Graphics* (Seattle, 1990). On Crimp see Timothy Druckrey, 'Douglas Crimp', *Flash Art* [international edition], CLI (1990), pp. 171–4. See also Alice Thorson, 'Visual AIDS II', *Afterimage*, XVIII (1990), p. 23; Lucy R. Lippard, 'Silence Still = Death', *High Performance*, XIV (1991), pp. 28–31.

14 See, for example, Pushpa Gupta and Kusum Kothari, 'Pretesting Communication Material', *Interaction*, VIII (1990), pp. 128–41; C. R. Evian, *et al.*, 'Qualitative Evaluation of an AIDS Education Poster: a Rapid Assessment Method for Health Education Materials', *South African Medical Journal*, LXXVIII (1990), pp. 517–20; J. P. Gardner, *et al.*, 'A HIV Information Poster for Display in Public Toilets', *International Conference on* AIDS, VIII (1992), abstract no. PuD 9072; O. Mueller, J. Lubega and J. Senoga, 'Knowledge and Attitude to Aids Shown by Ugandan School Children, Based On a Nationwide Poster Competition', *International Conference on* AIDS, V (1992), abstract no. W.E.P. 22.; G. Graves, 'Peer Participation in Poster Production', *International Conference on* AIDS, VI (1992), abstract no. F.D. 785.

15 Julia Kristeva, in her *Black Sun: Depression and Melancholia*, trans. Leon S. Roudiez (New York, 1989), describes Holbein's painting of the dead Christ as perhaps the first modern image of death: completely alien, as medieval death is not.

16 Elisabeth Bronfen, *Over her Dead Body: Death, Femininity and the Aesthetic* (New York, 1992).

17 Lee Edelman, 'The Plague of Discourse: Politics, Literary Theory, and AIDS', *South Atlantic Quarterly*, LXXXVIII (1989), pp. 302–17.

18 As in the images collected in Allen Ellenzweig, ed., *The Homerotic Photograph: Male Images from Durieu/Delacroix to Mapplethorpe* (New York, 1992).

19 Martti Grönfors and Olli Stålström, 'Power, Prestige, Profit: AIDS and the Oppression of Homosexual People', *Acta Sociologica*, XXX (1987), pp. 53–66, and Martin Eide, 'Dodskysset: Den Nye Nyheten om den Nye Pest', *Samtidem*, XCVIII (1989), pp. 6–12.

20 David L. Kirp and Ronald Bayer, eds, AIDS *in the Industrialized Democracies: Passions, Politics, and Policies* (New Brunswick, NJ, 1992).

21 Theodor Nasemann, AIDS: *Entwicklung einer Krankheit in Amerika und in Deutschland* (Stuttgart, 1987).

22 Compare Diane Richardson, *Women and the* AIDS *Crisis* (London, 1989).

23 Compare Michael Pollak, *The Second Plague of Europe:* AIDS *Prevention and Sexual Transmission among Men in Western Europe* (New York, 1993).

24 Dorothy Nelkin and Sander L. Gilman, 'Placing the Blame for Devastating Disease', in Arien Mack, ed., *In Time of Plague: The History and Social Consequences of Lethal Epidemic Disease* (New York, 1991), pp. 39–56.

25 Compare AIDS: *A Time to Care, A Time to Act: Towards a Strategy for Australians* (Canberra, 1988); Viva Gallego, 'Image, Myth and Metaphor in the AIDS Epidemic', *Australian Quarterly*, LX (1988), pp. 85–93.

26 Janice Zita Grover, 'Visible Lesions: Images of the PWA', *Afterimage*, XVII (1989), pp. 10–16.

27 These are reproduced throughout Frank Wagner, *op. cit.*

28 On my initial discussion of this theme see Sander L. Gilman, *Sexuality: An Illustrated History* (New York, 1989), pp. 319–21.

29 'Another Furor over a Benetton Ad', *The New York Times* (29 January 1992), section D, p. 17; Paula Span, 'Colored with Controversy: Outcry over Benetton Ad showing AIDS Deathbed Scene', *Washington Post* (13 February 1992), section D, p. 1. An analagous 'scandal' was generated by the use of images of the

mentally handicapped in British advertising: see 'Fuji Ad Sparks Disabled Media Images Debate', *British Journal of Photography*, CXXXIX (8 August 1991), p. 4.

30 Skip Wollenberg, 'Benetton Ads OK in US,' *Boston Globe* (14 February 1992), p. 81; Martha T. Moore, 'Benetton Ad Tests Hard Side of Reality', *USA Today* (14 February 1992), section B, p. 7.

31 Stuart Elliot, 'Brochure on AIDS is the Latest Departure from Benetton', *The New York Times* (29 April 1992), section D, p. 19.

32 Jeff Nunokawa, '"All the Sad Young Men"': AIDS and the Work of the Mourning', in Diane Fuss, ed., *Inside/Out, op. cit.*, pp. 311–23.

33 Sander L, Gilman, 'Touch, Sexuality and Disease', in William Bynum and Roy Porter, eds, *Medicine and the Five Senses* (Cambridge, 1993), pp. 198–224.

34 Frank Rich, 'The New Blood Culture', *The New York Times* (6 December 1992), section 9, p. 1.

Towards a Conclusion

1 See the selection of readings in Maurice Berger, ed., *Modern Art and Society: An Anthology of Social and Multicultural Readings* (New York, 1994).

2 In this context see the essays in C. Nadia Seremetakis, ed., *The Senses Still: Perception and Memory as Material Culture in Modernity* (Boulder, CO, 1994).

3 In general here see Slavoj Žižek, *The Sublime Object of Ideology* (London, 1989), pp. 87–130, and Ernesto Laclau and Chantal Mouffe, *Hegemony and Socialist Strategy; Towards a Radical Democratic Politics* (London, 1985), pp. 93–148.

4 James Hillman, *Interviews – Conversations with Laura Pozzo* (New York, 1983), p. 54.

5 See my essay on 'Touch, Sexuality and Disease' in William Bynum and Roy Porter, eds., *Medicine and the Five Senses* (Cambridge, 1993), pp. 98–224.

6 I want to thank Candice Breitz for her help during my stay in South Africa and following. Without her knowledge of the art scene, I would not have been able to orient myself as quickly as I did.

7 S. M. Johnson *et al.*, 'Student's Stereotypes of Patients as Barriers to Clinical Decision-making', *Journal of Medical Education*, LXI (1986), pp. 727–35.

Photographic Acknowledgements

The author and publishers wish to express their thanks to the following sources of illustrative material and/or permission to reproduce it: The National Library of Medicine, Bethesda, Maryland: illus. nos. 4–19, 21, 22, 25–27, 29–30, 33–77, 39–40, 42–46, 53–91; the Freud Museum, London: 51, 52; the Library, the Wellcome Institute for the History of Medicine, London: 28 (photo: © the Trustee of the Wellcome Trust); the Museum of Modern Art Photo Archive, New York: 31; the Pennsylvania Academy of the Fine Arts, Philadelphia: 13 (The Muriel and Philip Berman Gift acquired from the John S. Phillips bequest of 1876 to the Pennsylvania Academy of the Fine Arts, with funds contributed by Muriel and Philip Berman and the gifts (by exchange) of Lisa Norris Elkins, Bryant W. Langston and the Samuel S. White III and Vera White Collection, with additional funds (by exchange) given by Skelton Harrison and the Phillip H. and A. S. W. Rosenbach Foundation).

Index